THE
Vaccination
DEBATE

THE
Vaccination
DEBATE

Making the Right Choice for You and Your Children

CHRIS SPINELLI, DO, & MARYANN KARINCH

NEW HORIZON PRESS
Far Hills, New Jersey

Requests for permission should be addressed to:
New Horizon Press
P. O. Box 669
Far Hills, NJ 07931

Chris Spinelli, DO, and Maryann Karinch
The Vaccination Debate:
Making the Right Choice for You and Your Children

Cover design: Charley Nasta
Interior design: Scribe Inc.

Library of Congress Control Number: 2014957544

ISBN-13 (pb): 978–0-88282–505–2
ISBN-13 (eBook): 978–0-88282–506–9

New Horizon Press

Manufactured in the U.S.A.

19   18   17   16   15   1   2   3   4   5

Table of Contents

Introduction: A Genuine Vaccination Debate ix

Chapter 1: Is There Really a Problem with
Decreased Vaccinations? 1

Chapter 2: What Do Vaccines Do to an Infant or Toddler? . . . 21

Chapter 3: How Do Vaccines Affect Young Children
and Adolescents? 47

Chapter 4: How Do Vaccines Affect Adults of Any Age? 65

Chapter 5: The Autism Debate 77

Chapter 6: The Additives and Preservatives Debate 103

Chapter 7: The Natural Immunity Debate 119

Chapter 8: The Homeopathy Debate 135

Chapter 9: The Political Debate 149

Chapter 10: The Future of Vaccination Debates 167

Conclusion: Making Up Your Mind to Be
Pro- or Anti-Vaccine 193

Acknowledgments 195

Glossary 197

Endnotes 203

Index 225

Dedications

To my wife and children, whose support I greatly appreciate, plus the current and former members of the United States military. Thank you for all you've done for the citizens of our country and those around the world.

— Chris Spinelli

Thank you to my mother, whose high standards as a nurse and a parent put me on a good path from the start; to my brother, who helps me lighten up; and to Jim, who is there for me every day of every year.

— Maryann Karinch

To Rotary International, whose efforts to help eradicate polio worldwide have reduced the number of cases by 99 percent in the past thirty years.

— Chris and Maryann

A Genuine Vaccination Debate

Asked about whether vaccines for childhood diseases such as measles, mumps, rubella (MMR) and polio should be required or left up to parental choice, 68 percent of adults say such vaccines should be required while 30 percent say that parents should be able to decide whether or not to vaccinate their children.[1]

— Pew Research Center

When one-third of a population does not buy into the value of a common medical practice, it's time to air the science—all relevant parts of it—rather than throw the dissenters in jail, fine them or mock them in the media.

According to a website supported by The College of Physicians of Philadelphia (historyofvaccines.org), the Chinese introduced the first vaccine around 1000 CE. It was a smallpox inoculation (or variolation, as it was called at the time) and use of the smallpox material to prevent the disease spread to Africa and Turkey and then on to Europe and the Americas.

However, a friend of coauthor Maryann thinks the concept of using the source of illness to prevent or cure an illness can be tracked to an earlier time. The friend said, "Take a look at Numbers," which is one of the books of the Old Testament in the Bible. It could be argued that the passage about the healing power of a serpent-twined rod—one of several links to the symbol of modern medicine—also hints at the concept of vaccination. The upshot of the Prophet Moses' message, loosely translated, goes like this: "Don't worry about dying from a snake bite, because God made it possible for the snake I've got wrapped around this pole to save your life."

We can probably assume that there were both Chinese and Israelites who argued that what they were being told didn't make sense. Dissenters have been around for quite a while.

There have been dissenters in both the twentieth and twenty-first centuries, long before model Jenny McCarthy became an evangelist about a possible link between vaccinations and autism. A study published in the *Yale Journal of Biology and Medicine* spotlights references to vaccines in newspaper articles between 1915 and 1922 that call it "poisonous, filthy, loathsome, damnable stuff."[2] But with the aid of social media, disconnected pockets of parents against vaccination, or at least suspicious of it, were able to come together easily. Hence, the reason Eric Kodish, MD, a medical ethicist at the Cleveland Clinic, could assert in a June 26, 2014, *Washington Post* article that "The anti-vaccination movement is a relatively new one that has taken hold over the past decade."[3]

Regardless of who figured out that illnesses could be controlled or even eradicated through the use of "disease material," there are plenty of people who now think the concept is horrible. A violation of nature. A tool of the government to control people.

This book illuminates key arguments in the vaccination debate and states, with as much scientific power as possible, what drives the anti-vaccination contingent as well as what the pro-vaccination community stands on as evidence of the necessity of vaccinating our population.

We, the authors, believe that vaccines are some of the most important public health tools. At the same time, we are aware that people who don't agree want their arguments put into the context of a legitimate debate.

In this book, the debate encompasses the science behind and the science (when it exists) against each type of vaccine, as well as the timing of vaccinations, natural immunities, homeopathy and the use of heavy metals and other "additives."

We also look at the future of vaccinations. Currently, twenty vaccines are in common use and new techniques for developing vaccines give scientists hope of generating immunity against parasitic diseases such as malaria. Will humans one day have dozens of vaccines available so anyone with access to good medical care theoretically wouldn't have to worry about HIV, Ebola or even different kinds of cancer? The HIV vaccine has been in development for twenty years at this point and is in clinical trials, so this is more leading-edge medicine than futuristic medicine. But in the future, will only pediatricians, family practitioners, internists (who commonly administer the vaccines) and people like radiologists and orthopedic surgeons (who document and fix injuries that vaccines can't prevent) be nearly the only physicians with job security?

The vaccination debate is complicated.

Thirty percent of Americans and many more people worldwide have genuine concerns, fears or serious questions about vaccines. This book is meant to engage the questions, assertions and feelings of both sides so that a meaningful decision can be made as to what is best for both you and your children.

— *Chris Spinelli, DO, and Maryann Karinch*

CHAPTER 1

Is There Really a Problem with Decreased Vaccinations?

Are vaccines heroes or villains?

In this chapter we utilize a foundational discussion of disease prevention versus health risks. By health risks, we mean the health conditions that some people assert are *caused* by vaccines.

According to a poll conducted by the C.S. Mott Children's National Poll on Children's Health, 89 percent of the 1,621 parents who participated rated "vaccine safety" as the most important topic in children's health research today.[1]

The two other big topics were concerns about "things in the environment that could lead to health issues" and "new treatments for rare childhood diseases" at 72 percent and 66 percent, respectively.[2] Parents worry about their children getting sick, how to prevent illness and then how to take care of them when they do have health conditions.

Concerned parents like these are on both sides of the vaccination debate. They want to be proactive about their children's welfare.

Even though most parents in the United States willingly take their children to the doctor for the standard regimen of vaccinations designed by the Advisory Committee on Immunization Practices (ACIP) and endorsed by the American Academy of Pediatrics (AAP), the twenty-first century has seen a dramatic rise in the number of parents who do not. There is an even greater number who question the government-endorsed vaccination schedule, even though they comply completely or partially. According to the Mott report,

> In this Poll, parents overwhelmingly endorse the need for research on the safety of vaccines and medications given to children. Parental concerns about the safety of vaccines has increased markedly over the last decade, due to alleged (but later disproven) links between vaccines and autism and related concerns about mercury and other preservatives used in vaccines. For parents, assurances from healthcare providers and government officials that "vaccines are safe" have been insufficient. Rather, parents want more research about the safety of vaccines for their young children and adolescents.[3]

Clearly, as passionate as most pediatricians and family doctors are about getting their patients vaccinated, that passion does not allay the fears of many parents. There is just as much emotion on the other side. In this book we attempt to mute the emotion and turn up the volume on the facts. And so the debate begins.

First we will adopt the point of view that vaccines are "heroes" and then offer a set of countering arguments addressing some significant ways that vaccines might be portrayed as "villains."

VACCINES AS "HEROES"

Waste management is the most important factor in preventing disease and pestilence and remaining healthy. Certainly exercise and nutrition are good for you as well, but nothing trumps taking out the trash. So if taking out the trash is the best thing you can do to reduce disease on a civilization scale, what would the second best thing be?

The short answer from a lot of people is "vaccination," which many laud as the second-best public health initiative there is to reduce serious disease and illness. To take a close look at why that might stand as fact, let's consider what childhood afflictions are directly linked to environmental—as opposed to genetic—causes.

Today a lot of people don't realize what it's like to live in a country or an era where there are no vaccines. Those who have no visual or kinesthetic perception of what the vaccine-preventable diseases are like should spend a while in parts of the world where a lot of these diseases are rampant. In some countries, they are blunted due to the fact that some people do get vaccines; however, not everybody can be vaccinated as we can in the United States, so disease is still prevalent.

If you have had exposure to vaccine discussions before, you are aware that pro-vaxxers are constantly trying to win the vaccination debate by citing how many lives and dollars are saved through immunization programs. Nonetheless, a few numbers are important to make the case that vaccines have taken a huge bite out of the devastation caused by multiple infectious diseases—and that impact affects you personally. It affects your health and your flexibility in making certain choices about how to manage your children's health.

Starting with poliovirus, here is what the World Health Organization (WHO) says about this crippling disease in the world today:

Polio does still exist, although polio cases have decreased by over 99 percent since 1988, from an estimated more than 350,000 cases to 416 reported cases in 2013. This reduction is the result of the global effort to eradicate the disease. Today, only three countries in the world have never stopped transmission of polio (Nigeria, Pakistan and Afghanistan).

Despite the progress achieved since 1988, as long as a single child remains infected with poliovirus, children in all countries are at risk of contracting the disease. The poliovirus can easily be imported into a polio-free country and can spread rapidly among unimmunized populations. Failure to eradicate polio could result, within ten years, in as many as 200,000 new cases every year all over the world.

There is no cure for polio; it can only be prevented. Polio vaccine, given multiple times, can protect a child for life.[4]

According to the Centers for Disease Control and Prevention (CDC), between two and ten out of 100 people who are paralyzed by polio die because the virus affects the muscles that help them breathe.[5]

The Philippines has widespread cases of the measles, with 21,420 confirmed cases and 110 deaths in 2014, according to the CDC.[6] Syria, which had a 95 percent vaccination rate until 2010, had a 2013 vaccination rate of 45 percent because of the country's widespread violence.[7] As people flee across borders to find safety, they are taking measles or the vulnerability to measles along with them. Between February 9 and July 5, 2013, measles killed thirty-six people in Nigeria.[8] Even the "happiest place on earth"—Disneyland—became a third-world country in early 2015 when a measles outbreak eventually involving an estimated 188 people moved the vaccination debate into the headline news.[9]

Many people think of measles as a rash that's annoying, but you get over it. It's actually a highly contagious *respiratory disease* with a blotchy rash being just one symptom. "It's still one of the major killers in the developing world of kids under the age of five," according to Professor Gareth Williams, an authority on the history of vaccination and the author of *Angel of Death: The Story of Smallpox*, who also notes that 130,000 children a year still die of measles in India alone.[10] About 30 percent of measles victims develop complications, such as ear infections, pneumonia or encephalitis. It's unlikely that Jenny McCarthy, *Playboy* model and autism activist, had all the facts about deaths and complications from her research on vaccines—particularly the supposed link between the measles vaccine and autism—when she stated on CNN: "You ask any mother in the autism community and we'll take the flu, the measles over autism any friggin' day of the week."[11]

If every child is, indeed, as unique as often asserted by people who feel that vaccines are not right for their children, consider the case of Emmalee Parker. She was distinctive. Only seven people in a million who ever contract measles experience a case as unusual as hers.

Born in India, Emmalee was adopted by a Philadelphia area couple. The paperwork took over a year, so by the time her adoptive parents got Emmalee to the United States, she was two-and-a-half years old. She seemed to have both health and behavior problems, so her parents took her to various specialists. Five years after adoption, she started losing coordination, which resulted in a trip to the Children's Hospital of Philadelphia. The emergency room physicians there who were from India asked when she had had the measles. They recognized Emmalee's symptoms as a rare measles complication called Subacute Sclerosing Panencephalitis (SSPE).

SSPE results from a defective form of the measles virus replicating in the nervous system. The child has a persistent infection that causes a series of problems before the patient typically dies: mental deterioration, loss of muscle control, seizures and muscle twitching. The onset of symptoms might be years after the person first contracted measles; in fact, it's occurred as many as twenty-seven years later.[12]

Emmalee slipped into a coma a few months after that visit to the emergency room. She died a month after her eighth birthday.

The lesson is not just that there are horrible complications of measles—no matter how rare they are. It's that Emmalee wasn't vaccinated at the right time. In the orphanage in India, she received the measles vaccine at sixteen months: "The Parkers were told that it is likely that she got SSPE because she was exposed to measles before she was one year old."[13]

As a prelude to the debate in chapter 3 about the vaccine schedule, we'll note here that the first dose of the measles vaccine is usually given at nine months in the United States as part of the MMR (measles/mumps/rubella) injection. The primary alternative schedule developed by pediatrician Robert W. Sears and specified in *The Vaccine Book* calls for this vaccine to be administered at the one-year mark.[14] The success of vaccinations in controlling and eradicating disease involves the science of antigens and the science of timing.

Critics of vaccines may want to take a look at this list of the top ten infectious diseases and how many are either currently preventable with vaccines or likely to be preventable due to emerging vaccines, such as live recombinant vaccines, which hold hope for prevention of AIDS. Keep in mind that infectious disease is the world's biggest killer of children and young adults.

Most of us don't have anything to worry about with anthrax, while smallpox was officially eradicated in 1977 thanks to vaccines. But military personnel do receive immunizations from some of these deadly infectious diseases, because either the disease exists where the military is going or the disease has been weaponized—as in the case of anthrax.

Until June 2014, we could have also said that most of us don't have anything to worry about with bubonic plague. Then

TABLE I: TOP TEN INFECTIOUS DISEASES[15]	
DISEASE (IN REVERSE ORDER)	PREVENTABLE BY VACCINE
10. Influenza (Flu)	Yes
9. HIV/AIDS	Working on it
8. Tuberculosis (TB)	Yes
7. Anthrax	Yes
6. Cholera	Yes
5. MRSA	Working on it
4. Rabies	Yes
3. Smallpox	Yes
2. Bubonic Plague	Yes
1. Ebola	Working on it

Compiled from public reports issued by the Centers for Disease Control and Prevention and the World Health Organization

a Colorado man ended up in the hospital with a horrible lung infection that doctors couldn't seem to diagnose. One of the physicians sent a sample to the state health laboratory and a team there determined he was infected with pneumonic plague, a first cousin to bubonic plague—the cause of the Black Death in Europe during the Middle Ages. Three other people then got it. Suddenly, a disease that American doctors had never seen and one that many Americans would have probably said was either eradicated or impossible to find in the United States made a dramatic appearance.

After a great deal of investigation, it was determined the man caught the disease from his pet pit bull terrier, who had most likely gotten it from a prairie dog. Two of the other people who got the plague at that time had worked in the veterinary clinic where the dog was treated. The third infected person had been around the infected man and his dog. Her case signified the first airborne transmission of plague in the United States in ninety years.[16]

TABLE 2: KEY NOTIFIABLE DISEASES IN
THE UNITED STATES: PROFILE OF CHANGING RATES

	DISEASE	NEW CASES IN 1960	NEW CASES IN 2000	NEW CASES IN 2010
1.	Sexually transmitted diseases (does not include HIV/AIDS)	503,527	1,135,902	1,708,946
2.	Salmonellosis (infection caused by Salmonella; food poisoning)	6,929	39,574	54,424
3.	Lyme disease	unreported	17,730	30,158
4.	**Pertussis (whooping cough)**	**14,809**	**7,867**	**27,550**
5.	Shigellosis (infection caused by Shigella; food poisoning)	12,487	22,922	14,786
6.	**Tuberculosis**	**55,494**	**16,377**	**11,182**
7.	**Hepatitis B**	**8,310**	**8,036**	**3,374**
8.	**Haemophilus influenza (Hib)**	**unreported**	**13,397**	**3,151**
9.	**Mumps**	**100,000+**[17]	**338**	**2,612**
10.	Rocky Mountain Spotted Fever	unreported	495	1,985
11.	**Hepatitis A**	**55,000+**[18]	**13,397**	**1,670**
12.	**Meningoccocal disease (meningitis)**	**2,500+**[19]	**2,256**	**833**

Compiled from public reports issued by the Centers for Disease Control and Prevention and the World Health Organization

Despite our continuing vulnerabilities, isn't it a comfort to look at the list and know that nearly all of the main infectious diseases in the world are preventable?

It's useful to take another look at the top infectious diseases to show which ones are the biggest threats in the United States; it's very different from the infectious disease threats to low-income and developing nations.

Table 2 is populated by statistics on "notifiable diseases," which refers to diseases that must be reported to government authorities. Some of them, like salmonellosis (a type of food poisoning) and Lyme disease, are clearly not in the category of contagious diseases like measles or mumps, but they took their place on the table of the top twelve as of 2010.[20] As you might expect, measles and tuberculosis used to be very high in the rankings before the introduction of vaccines combating them, but they've since been replaced by diseases such as those caused by bad bacteria in a food source and deer ticks.

We compare the numbers of new cases in 1960, 2000 and 2010 in order to see the impact of vaccines on the occurrence of certain diseases. The diseases addressed by vaccines and their related statistics are bolded.

Of particular note is that it's easy to see the rise in cases of certain preventable illnesses after the anti-vaccination movement started picking up steam in the United States and Canada in the early twenty-first century. At that point, more parents decided to do selective vaccinations, meaning they might forego the measles/mumps/rubella (MMR) and pertussis (whooping cough) immunization, but they would agree to a shot to combat diphtheria. For this reason, you can see a rise in measles/mumps/rubella and pertussis cases between 2000 and 2010, but the number of diphtheria cases—not even on this top twelve chart—dropping from 918 in 1960 to zero by 2010.

Critics of vaccines are quick to make their arguments personal by using compelling anecdotes to counter the pro-vaccine community's impressive statistics. So here's a pro-vaccination anecdote reported in *The Denver Post* on April 16, 2015 to accent the statistics:

A Canadian woman who had declined to have her children immunized against pertussis, better known as whooping cough, has changed her position now that all seven of her children have come down with the disease.

Tara Hills was stuck in isolation at her Ottawa home for more than a week with her sick children. Whooping cough, a bacterial infection, causes violent, uncontrollable coughing and is best known for the telltale sound victims make as they try to draw breath. Occasionally, it can be fatal, especially in infants less than a year old, according to the Centers for Disease Control and Prevention.[21]

The story also noted that Canada has had declining vaccination rates in some communities just as the United States has seen a drop. Hills' reason for having partially vaccinated her first three children and then abandoning vaccinations completely with her four youngest is a statement that invites compassion—and criticism of the websites that offer only anecdotes or misinformation: "We stopped because we were scared and didn't know who to trust."[22]

Another statistic worth noting to show the impact of vaccinations and avoidance of vaccinations: In 1960, there were 441,703 cases of Rubeola (measles). That number dropped to a low point of sixty-three in 2010, but then shot up to 220 by 2011. There have been no more reported cases of diphtheria since 2000 (when there was just one) and only one reported case of polio since 2000.

If you are duly impressed by the small number of cases of deadly diseases such as tuberculosis, measles, whooping cough and meningitis, consider what would happen if we stopped our immunization programs that keep the numbers low. Bottom line: We would be at risk for dramatic increases, like the January 2015 measles outbreak that began in Disneyland hinted at.

A critical factor to consider is that certain diseases work very quickly, so without immunization they will result in major damage or death. Basically, treatment often can't catch up with the disease, much less overtake it. That's the case with meningococcal disease, which can leave you dead in six hours.

In the rest of the world, the annual infection rates for these diseases are as captured in the following table.

TABLE 3: INFECTION RATES GLOBALLY FOR KEY VACCINE-PREVENTABLE DISEASES		
DISEASE	ANNUAL MORTALITY RATE	ANNUAL INFECTION RATE
Tuberculosis	2 million	8 million
Measles	530,000	30 million
Whooping cough	200,000–300,000	20–40 million
Meningitis	174,000	1 million+

Compiled from public reports issued by the Centers for Disease Control and Prevention and the World Health Organization

Overall we have done a great job of targeting serious, highly contagious diseases with vaccines. A specific success of vaccines would be smallpox: We don't see smallpox anymore unless it is in a laboratory that has been working with it or in a movie in which art imitates life and the disease has been weaponized.

Before the official eradication of smallpox—the last naturally occurring case was in Somalia in 1977—the general population received smallpox inoculations just like most of us get the MMR and other shots as kids. In 1983, distribution of smallpox vaccine to the general civilian population was discontinued, but the threat of smallpox becoming a bioterror weapon has caused the United States to inoculate special populations. The result has been an unhappy one for some people.

Between January 24 and March 28, 2003, a total of 29,584 civilian health-care and public health workers received a smallpox vaccine as part of an effort to prepare US personnel for a potential terrorist attack involving the smallpox virus. There were ten cardiac adverse events reported among the civilian recipients; there were also cases of heart-related issues among the military recipients. However, the only serious one involved a pre-existing condition exacerbated by smoking.[23]

The trouble with the most recent smallpox vaccine rollout was that, in general, Americans have become heavier and less conditioned than the previous generations that received the vaccine. When the vaccine seemed to increase heart inflammation/problems, it was hard to tell if it was really the vaccine or just our poor health. Ultimately, the smallpox vaccine was discontinued for civilian use, but it is still used for military personnel today. Individuals in the military are typically not fat and the reported heart inflammation rates were 0.012 percent for military and 0.085 percent for civilians. The military people also had a very high rate of quick recovery after their reported post-vaccination incidents.

The purpose of mentioning the adverse reactions to the "heroic" smallpox vaccine is that populations change and sometimes we see either new effects or coincidental occurrences in relation to medications and foods. Although it will be discussed in much greater depth in chapter 5 on the autism debate, we're setting the stage now by referencing that there may be a number of changing environmental and genetic factors that can influence how such "heroic" vaccines are perceived by a new generation.

VACCINES AS "VILLAINS"

Smallpox was one of the world's most devastating and disgusting diseases. The Chinese developed an inoculation for it around the year 1000 CE, but it wasn't until the mid-to-late eighteenth

century that aggressive measures were taken to protect populations. It was mandatory that members of the Continental Army
receive inoculations against smallpox. Certainly, there have always
been people who questioned the safety of the vaccine, which
evolved as research became more sophisticated, but smallpox was
such an ugly disease that it was easy to hate and the impetus was
to take even desperate measures to protect against it. Side effects?
Who cared, if you could avoid getting smallpox!

Fortunately, by the twenty-first century other devastating
diseases like diphtheria and polio joined the zero incidence rate
in the United States. Most recently, in late April of 2015, the
Pan American Health Organization (PAHO) announced that the
Western Hemisphere was officially free of rubella (or German
measles). One can argue credibly that, at least in some pockets
of the country, herd immunity exists for measles, mumps and
possibly a few other vaccine-preventable diseases as well. Herd
immunity is generally defined in terms of 90–95 percent of a
population being immune to a particular contagious disease, pre-
sumably through vaccination.

This shift in danger levels facing people of all ages is one
of the contributing factors to a re-evaluation of vaccine safety
by many people. Without the imminent risk of contracting a
debilitating or deadly disease, the willingness to accept reassur-
ances that a substance made up of multiple chemicals as well as
some kind of virus or bacteria is harmless has diminished. Jim
McCormick, founder and president of the Research Institute for
Risk Intelligence, sums up the change in attitude this way: "Risk
inclination is situational. It varies based on the circumstances
with which we're presented."[24]

Another contributing factor is the ability of individuals
around the world to connect with each other and share anecdotes and opinions. A father in New York whom we spoke with
has actively used social media, op-eds and articles to discuss the

onset of his daughter's autism symptoms after her MMR vaccination; instead of being a parent alone with a story, there are now many thousands of people who know about his experience and have shared their own as well.

The combination of (a) no perception of imminent threat from deadly disease with (b) a convergence of real stories of very young children suddenly "changing" has created momentum to investigate the possible side effects of vaccines and to resist the prescribed "government-endorsed" schedule.

The critics who pride themselves on a combination of empirical evidence and some knowledge of science—those who think that at least some vaccines are "villains" to certain people in the population—ask a powerful and worthwhile question: Should what we're doing today with immunizations be the same as what we did yesterday? And by "yesterday," they don't mean the mid-twentieth century when smallpox, polio and diphtheria were still threats. They mean a decade ago or less.

Many people we spoke with are not critical of all vaccinations, but they wonder who is doing what to boost their safety so that "little risk" hopefully becomes "no risk." And as the Mott poll suggests, many do not believe that there is adequate ongoing research about vaccine safety.

Suzanne Humphries, MD, is a nephrologist specializing in kidney disease and treatment. An outspoken critic of vaccines, Humphries is also one of the few who has fled the medical establishment after becoming convinced that vaccines—some more than others—are "villains." Despite the fact that she has been heavily criticized after her disavowal of traditional Western medicine, Humphries references a few credible studies on her website. These studies suggest that some scientists are questioning the general perception of two things: first, that vaccines always do what they are supposed to do and second, that ill effects from them are rare.

One of the studies Humphries references was conducted by a team of researchers who published their findings in *Clinical Infectious Diseases*, a peer-reviewed journal published by Oxford University Press. The title captures their interesting findings: "Increased risk of non-influenza respiratory virus infections associated with receipt of inactivated influenza vaccine."

The team randomly selected a group of 115 children aged six to fifteen whose parents allowed them to participate in a double-blind study in which neither the subjects nor the research team knew which children got a flu vaccine and which ones got a placebo. They followed the health situation of all these children for nine months after the flu vaccine or placebo had been administered. Their study ultimately led to an enigmatic result and the researchers so much as said, "We don't know why this would happen." Their highly technical summary of possibilities suggested potential reporting errors, factors related to exposure to certain diseases in the community and a few other things. But the research team also stated succinctly what else they thought could be a distinct possibility:

> The increased risk could also indicate a real effect. Receipt of TIV [trivalent inactivated influenza vaccine] could increase influenza immunity at the expense of reduced immunity to non-influenza respiratory viruses, by some unknown biological mechanism.[25]

From a vaccine critic's point of view, the argument gets even better. The study also states, "There was no statistically significant difference in the risk of confirmed seasonal influenza infection between recipients of TIV or placebo."[26]

Keep in mind that this was a small study. Even so, the research methods described in the paper seem both sound and well-documented, including the fact that serum specimens were drawn from the subjects before vaccination so the team had base-line information. Combined with the nine-month follow-up, the study suggests at the very least that similar research should be conducted. With decent research, there is often an open door to other research.

Given that most of the really serious accusations about the health hazards of vaccines address neurological disorders, it is important to look at studies that examine this correlation spe-cifically. First, we want to present a list of the disorders that are targeted by Joseph Mercola, an osteopathic physician and pro-ponent of alternative medicine, who operates a well-trafficked "health information" site.

Mercola unequivocally views vaccines as "villains," choosing instead to endorse supplements and homeopathic approaches to strengthening immunity. It should also be noted that Mercola received warnings from the US Food and Drug Administration (FDA) in 2005, 2006 and 2011—a total of seven warnings that were related to products sold on his website and another set of warnings about the misrepresentation of a diagnostic tool; that's relevant because these warnings were related to what the FDA deemed unsubstantiated claims of the value of his supplements and the diagnostic tool.[27] Nonetheless, Mercola has a very large fol-lowing and has made repeated appearances on the *Dr. Oz Show*—an implied endorsement from the popular Dr. Mehmet Oz.

Mercola's List of Vaccination-induced Neurological Disorders[28]

- Apraxia (a speech disorder)
- Ataxia (a lack of muscle control during voluntary movements, such as walking)
- Auto-immune Diseases (such as lupus, Crohn's disease and eczema, among others)
- Blindness

- Brain tumors/SV-40 (This one makes no sense today, but it adds an interesting historical note. According to the Mayo Clinic: "...Simian virus 40 (SV40) [is] a virus originally found in monkeys. Millions of people may have been exposed to SV40 when receiving polio vaccinations between 1955 and 1963, because the vaccine was developed using monkey cells. Once it was discovered that SV40 was linked to certain cancers, the virus was removed from the polio vaccine."[29])
- Convulsions (seizures)
- Deafness
- Demyelinating diseases (any nervous system disease in which the nerve coating is damaged)
- Encephalitis (an inflammation of the brain)
- Epilepsy
- Guillain-Barré Syndrome (a rare disorder in which the body's immune system attacks the nerves)
- Hyperactivity—ADD/ADHD, LD (Attention Deficit Disorder/ Attention Deficit Hyperactivity Disorder, Learning Disabilities)
- Lupus (a chronic inflammatory disease that occurs when a body's immune system attacks that body's own tissues and organs)
- Meningitis Paralysis
- Mental confusion (lowered IQ)
- Multiple Sclerosis (similar to Guillain-Barré Syndrome, MS is a disease in which the immune systems attacks the protective covering on the nerves)
- Paralytic polio
- Retardation
- Sudden Infant Death Syndrome (SIDS)

A literature search suggests that much of Mercola's list emerged from a combination of anecdotal evidence, historical (not current) facts and studies done on rabies vaccines in the late 1980s. Research supporting Mercola's specific assertions would include:

- A 1988 study published in *Neurology* entitled "Immunologic studies of rabies vaccination-induced Guillain-Barré syndrome"
- A 1989 study published in the *Journal of Neurological Sciences* entitled "Anticardiolipin antibodies in patients with rabies vaccination induced neurological complications and other neurological diseases"
  - o The specific "neurological complications" mentioned are these disorders, all of which are on Mercola's list: encephalitis, Guillain-Barré syndrome and Multiple Sclerosis (MS).
  - o There was also a non-committal statement about systemic lupus.

Rather than rely on these rabies vaccine studies, probably the most compelling support for people who believe vaccines can cause neurological damage comes from more modern—and balanced—research. One such study is "Vaccines and Neurologic Disease," the product of a pro-vaccination physician; however, this study cites documentation of a correlation in some cases between immunization and the onset of neurological problems.

Even to a pro-vaxxer, a vaccine is sometimes a "villain."

In the paper just referenced, published in *Seminars in Neurology* in 2011, James J. Sejvar, MD, notes:

Vaccines have undoubtedly decreased global morbidity and mortality from several infectious diseases by immeasurable amounts. The contributions of vaccines to global improvements in public health cannot be questioned. However, the nature of the mechanism by which vaccines afford protection through stimulation of the immune system results in the fact that, in rare circumstances, adverse events may follow vaccination.[30]

Sejvar also notes that a study with monkeys indicated how "a vaccine or vaccine proteins could directly damage the membranes of myelin or axons."[31] Myelin is a material that covers nerves and an axon is a nerve fiber, so this assertion tracks with some of the potential neurological disorders on Mercola's list.

As hard as either side might try to remain bulletproof, it's not going to happen when real science becomes a central part of the debate. One thing both sides can agree on is this: The research must be guided by inquiry, rather than by an agenda.

CHAPTER 2

What Do Vaccines Do to an Infant or Toddler?

et's look at the vaccines given to newborns through fifteen
months. This is the first age grouping in the schedule pro-
moted by the American Academy of Pediatrics (AAP) and Advisory
Committee on Immunization Practices (ACIP), whose recommen-
dations are official positions of the CDC. We will provide insights
into why they determined the vaccines should be given on this
schedule. We will also offer some historical perspective on the
targeted diseases and vaccines as well.

VACCINE AT BIRTH

Just after birth, an injection of hepatitis B vaccine is given to the
newborn. The aim is to reduce transmission of hepatitis B, which is a
liver infection, from mother to infant—and it must be given shortly
after birth to accomplish that. There is a 90–95 percent reduction in
transmission if it is given to vulnerable infants at this early stage.

Administering the vaccine at birth has been a recommendation from the CDC since 1991, which is five years after the

development of a second generation of the vaccine. Before that, a vaccine derived from plasma had been used; blood from hepatitis B virus-infected donors went through processing to make the virus inactive. In contrast, the second-generation vaccine that was developed in 1986 and is now used on newborns results from genetic engineering. It's synthetically prepared and does not contain blood products, so it's impossible to get hepatitis B from the new DNA recombinant vaccines that are currently in use in the United States.[1]

Vaccinating newborns may seem too severe until you know how likely it is that a new mother has hepatitis B—and that many people don't know they have it:

> Worldwide, two billion people [that's about one out of 3.5 people currently on the planet] have been infected with hepatitis B. Four hundred million people have become chronically infected (which means they are unable to get rid of the virus). An estimated one million people die each year from hepatitis B and its complications.
>
> In the United States, over twelve million people have been infected (that's one out of twenty people). Almost 100,000 new people are infected with hepatitis B each year. An estimated 5,000 Americans die each year from hepatitis B and its complications.[2]

People other than babies get hepatitis B through unprotected sex, sharing or re-using needles and exposure to the blood of an infected person. Newborns get hepatitis B during delivery from an infected mother as they leave the protection of the womb and placenta and are exposed to the mother's blood and body fluids. Unvaccinated infants who are exposed to hepatitis B have a 90 percent chance of becoming chronic carriers of the disease. Of those infected, a quarter of them will eventually develop Hep B-related

BIRTH TO FIFTEEN MONTHS

VACCINE	BIRTH	1 MO	2 MOS	4 MOS	6 MOS	9 MOS	12 MOS	15 MOS
Hepatitis B (Hep B)	←1st dose→	←2nd dose→			←3rd dose→			
Rotavirus (RV) RV1 (2-dose series); RV5 (3-dose series)			←1st dose→	←2nd dose→	←3rd dose→			
Diphtheria, tetanus, & acellular pertussis (DTaP: <7 yrs)			←1st dose→	←2nd dose→	←3rd dose→			←4th dose→
Haemophilus influenzae type b (Hib)			←1st dose→	←2nd dose→			←3rd or 4th dose→	
Pneumococcal conjugate (PCV13)			←1st dose→	←2nd dose→	←3rd dose→		←4th dose→	
Inactivated poliovirus (IPV; <18 yrs)			←1st dose→	←2nd dose→		←3rd dose→		
Influenza (IIV; LAIV)					Annual vaccination (IIV only) 1 or 2 doses			
Measles, mumps, rubella (MMR)							←1st dose→	
Varicella (VAR)							←1st dose→	
Hepatitis A (Hep A)							←2 dose series→	

liver cancer or cirrhosis. They have a 300–400 times greater risk of liver cancer if acquired this way.

Despite this preventable transmission, about five hundred infants a year still acquire the infection from their mothers at birth. This could happen because the mother was never tested due to little or no prenatal care; conversely, the mother may have had excellent prenatal care but acquired the infection during pregnancy after the initial test was completed and did not know about it. There are also the complications of results interpretation and test inaccuracy; errors like that may not happen often, but they do happen.

These testing-related issues are partially why many physicians take issue with Robert W. Sears, author of *The Vaccine Book* and the pediatrician who suggests one alternative is to only give the vaccine to newborns of hepatitis B-positive mothers.[3] Another reason they disagree with Sears: the possibility of infection from hepatitis B-positive individuals (other than the mother) who live in the household and will come into physical contact with the newborn.

The rationale for skipping the dose because the child "will get it at two months" doesn't work. If you're going to give it, give it at birth *and* at two months *and* six months. The reason for this timing is that chronic infection is more common in infants and children than adults. Infected people who don't appear sick can spread the virus to unvaccinated infants through contact with blood or other body fluids via breaks in the skin, such as bites, cuts, sores or contact with objects that can have fluids on them, such as toothbrushes.

VACCINES AT TWO MONTHS

Although the baby receives an initial hepatitis B inoculation at birth, the schedule calls for another injection at two months and then one again at six months. There are other vaccines that are recommended at their two-month appointment and this is where pediatricians and family doctors really start the childhood immunization process. Usually at two months, the child receives vaccinations for diphtheria, tetanus, pertussis, polio, *Haemophilus influenzae B* (Hib), pneumococcal disease and rotavirus, in addition to the shot for Hep B. It sounds like the medical version of encasing a baby in bubble wrap—and in a way, it is!

In many cases, the physician gives a single injection that combines five vaccines (diphtheria, tetanus, pertussis, Hep B and polio) called DTaP-Hep B-IPV; the brand name given to this vaccination by GlaxoSmithKline is Pediarix. However, there are stand-alone shots, as well as other types of combinations and brands. One example is Pentacel, manufactured by Sanofi Pasteur, which integrates vaccines for all of these cited except hepatitis B; instead, it includes protection against Hib.

If a parent wants nothing to do with Hep B, Hib or the IPV vaccine for polio, but wants protection against diphtheria, tetanus and pertussis, there are other combination vaccines for that option as well: Infanrix (GlaxoSmithKline), Daptacel or Tripedia (Sanofi Pasteur). There is also a version of Infanrix that is termed "preservative free."

Even more variations of the vaccines also exist today, so if a parent without a background in medicine or organic chemistry tried to make the decision based on independent research, it could be a daunting task.

DTAP: (DIPHTHERIA, TETANUS AND ACELLULAR PERTUSSIS)

Diphtheria infection causes a thick covering in the back of the throat that can lead to breathing problems, paralysis, heart failure and death.

The United States is among a number of nations with zero reported cases of diphtheria for several years. Given that reality, is Robert Sears right when he asserts in *The Vaccine Book*, "This illness is so rare that I put the risk at close to zero for all age groups?"[4] Yes and no—and the "no" part of that answer is why children still receive the diphtheria vaccine today.

If you look at a world map displaying cases of diphtheria, you'll see that if the North American countries of Canada and the United States closed their borders to everyone except most of Western Europe and a few other countries (those countries would have to do the same), then maybe we could forgo the diphtheria shot. But if you had to travel to India, Indonesia, Sudan or Iran—or if you had an infected traveler come near you—you'd be vulnerable at any age without the vaccine. The World Health Organization states that India alone reported 6,094 cases of diphtheria in 2014—that's 83 percent of the cases reported worldwide.[5]

Tetanus induces painful tightening of muscles all over the body. Caused by the toxin of a common bacterium, it's actually a nerve disorder. According to WebMD, the toxin behind tetanus ranks with botulism toxin as one of the most potent and "Once tetanus has spread, the mortality rate is approximately 30 percent, even in modern medical facilities."[6]

Because Sears' book and alternative schedule for (or suggestions on skipping) certain vaccinations has enjoyed such popularity, we are returning to his determination of the relative risks of tetanus. He says to his readers, "This disease is virtually unheard of in the first five years of life. We see only about ten cases annually among those who are between ages five and twenty-five, giving us a disease risk of only about one in 500,000."[7] Current statistics provided at the WebMD website suggest that his numbers are correct, but with a caveat: This was not the case before "Childhood immunization laws were passed in the United States in the 1970s."[8] An estimated one million infants still die of tetanus in developing countries each year; they are the victims of poor hygiene and lack of vaccination.

That makes the tetanus vaccine at two months for a baby in North America sound rather unnecessary—as long as you keep your baby in a Hazmat Onesie, since the bacterial spores that pose a risk can come from a bite from the family cat or dog, an insect bite, a splinter, dirt and other environmental risks.

Pertussis (whooping cough) is an infection that can result in coughing spells so severe that it's hard for the infant to eat, drink or even breathe. The infection can lead to pneumonia, seizures, brain damage and death. Worldwide, there are twenty to forty million pertussis cases and about 300,000 deaths per year. The United States had over 35,000 cases in 2012, with sixteen deaths. If you refer to Table 2 in chapter 1, you will see that the number of cases is steadily rising, up from 27,500 in 2010. The increase from an annual low of 1,730 in 1980 is considered by public health officials and the medical community to be directly attributable to the drop in the vaccination rate.

Around 40 percent of the time it's the mother who gives an infant pertussis, according to the CDC. Particularly for children four months and younger, fathers and other caregivers, as well as siblings and others who might be visitors to the household, are the other main source of the infection. There is also risk from the child's community, but it's considered small by comparison. Statistics like this indicate that keeping the baby home doesn't prevent all serious illnesses.[9]

There is currently a push to re-vaccinate the adult and adolescent population, because of the typical nature of transmission. The plan includes vaccinating mothers after birth and adding pertussis vaccine to the tetanus booster in adolescence. Both parties are often the ones that expose infants to these diseases and immunity to pertussis and tetanus, among other diseases, wanes over time.

As with all diseases covered by DTaP, the two-, four- and six-month doses are aimed at creating what we'd call "significant immunity." Regarding the repeat administration of many vaccines, not just DTaP, immunity is like exercise: You can't do it one time and say, "I'm done. That made me fit." Your immune system needs to be "exercised." In the short term, the vaccinations given to babies are designed to jumpstart the process of strengthening immunity, but the process is supposed to go on over the course of a person's life. Immune system resilience can also be affected by lifestyle choices, so get your booster shots!

Can you expect your baby to have a negative reaction to the vaccine? Actually, you should know how common it is for infants to have some degree of upset. DTaP vaccines can induce fevers. But then, nearly all vaccines can induce fever since they rev up the immune system and fever is a feature of that immune system. DTaP causes fever in 25 percent of children who receive the vaccine. We also see some tiredness and mild fussiness, typically the evening after vaccination. About 2 percent of children also experience some vomiting.[10]

Uncommon events reported are seizures in one in 14,000 children and high fever over 105 degrees in one in 16,000 children. To put this into perspective, the risk of Cystic Fibrosis in a Caucasian is one in 2,500. The risk of Cystic Fibrosis in an African American is one in 18,000.[11] And the risk of Muscular Dystrophy for anyone is one in 3,500.[12] Any of these events is sad, but all of them are uncommon. Exceptionally rare reports, which are hard to link directly to the vaccine since it's uncertain if we're seeing causality or coincidence, are long-term seizures, coma and brain damage. The reason it's difficult to link these to the vaccine is this: The typical person's seizure risk is 1 percent or one in 100, but the number we see after this vaccination is so far removed from that level that it could be the innate risk to blame for the seizure and not the vaccine. Some people believe otherwise, but you should think about this: If somebody has a family history of heart disease and is eating bacon-wrapped meatloaf and has a heart attack, what caused it? Would you say it was that high-fat food choice or family genetics? One could argue both.

HAEMOPHILUS INFLUENZAE B VACCINE

Haemophilus influenzae used to cause up to a reported 25 percent of US hospital admissions in the early 1980s before the vaccine was released. At that time, 20,000 children under five years of age got severe Hib disease each year and about 1,000 died annually.[13] So in the 1970s and part of the next decade, up to 25 percent of the kids who were admitted to the hospital were suffering from this one particular bacteria family. Meningitis was significant and severe, causing shock, sepsis (bacteria in the blood) and death. In fact, this illness caused a significant amount of death, including fatalities from epiglottitis, an inflammation and swelling of the tissue above the windpipe that prevents breathing. This illness typically hits children under five years of age the hardest.

There's good news and bad news with Hib. The good news relates to children. According to the CDC and recent studies, "Since the introduction of the *Haemophilus influenzae* type b vaccine, the incidence of invasive *H. influenzae* type b disease among children has fallen dramatically."[14] However, that's not the case for adults, as indicated by the data from Table 2 in chapter 1. Any assertion of herd immunity with something like Hib falls apart quickly in the face of these rising numbers in the population at large.

Coauthor Chris works with a family whose father is deaf from *Haemophilus influenzae* meningitis. The father cannot ever hear his child's voice or hear him call out "I love you, dad" due to the infection. He will never hear the sound of his child breathing peacefully at night. Later on, they will be able to communicate once the child learns sign language, but the father still misses out on many other things that parents enjoy in a child.

Side effects of Hib vaccine are typically fever, which may exceed 101 degrees in one out of twenty kids. In addition, local swelling and redness are always possible because, as we said before, vaccines rev up the immune system.

PNEUMOCOCCAL VACCINE

Pneumococcal disease is the leading cause of serious illness throughout the world, according to the National Foundation for Infectious Diseases. At fault is a common type of bacteria called the pneumococcus, which has the ability to attack different parts of the body and cause ear infections, pneumonias, sinusitis, sepsis, shock and meningitis. When kids get significant pneumococcal illnesses we are often able to treat them enough to save their lives with antibiotics and machines like respirators, but often they have left-over problems and are either physically or neurologically impaired for life.

The vaccine that we use for pneumococcal disease at the two-month appointment is Prevnar, which is manufactured by Wyeth Pharmaceuticals. There's a counterpart to it made by Merck for children over two years old and adults (mostly over fifty) that's called Pneumovax. Prevnar is similar to Pneumovax—the "pneumonia shot" that elderly people get—but Pneumovax has twenty-three subtypes in it, whereas Prevnar holds only thirteen. This vaccine can be given to two-month-olds and elicit the intended response, whereas the one with twenty-three subtypes does not generate the desired response in babies. (There is a current campaign to vaccinate adults over fifty with the Prevnar 13 as well.)

In early 2000, invasive pneumococcal disease caused about 200 deaths annually in kids under five years of age and was the leading cause of meningitis in the United States. For that reason, Sears' risk analysis seems cavalier: "Pneumococcus is a very common germ, yet most cases are fairly mild."[15]

At least 13,000 blood infections, 700 meningitis cases and five million ear infections were reported from this type of bacteria.

Children under two years of age are at the highest risk, but the previous vaccine for this organism didn't have much efficacy for children under two. An important side note is that pneumococcal infections are bacteria that currently have a high amount of resistance to the antibiotics commonly taken. It's a great argument for prevention whenever possible, since the antibiotics on which we rely so heavily may have limited effectiveness with this bug.

Current studies show a highly reduced prevalence in sepsis and bacteremia in the young infant from these bacteria now that the latest vaccine has been in use.

Downsides are possible side effects, which are similar to those of the Hib vaccine: one in fifty cases had a fever over 102.2 degrees and some of the children had localized redness and swelling.

POLIO VACCINE

The disease polio calls to mind a lot of high-profile people and a lot of heart-wrenching stories. Here are just some of the famous individuals who helped make the cry for a polio vaccine strong and loud:

- Franklin D. Roosevelt, 32nd president of the United States
- Donald Sutherland, Canadian-born actor
- Arthur C. Clarke, British science fiction writer
- Jack Nicklaus, legendary golfer known as "The Golden Bear"
- Mia Farrow, American actress
- Neil Young, Canadian singer/songwriter
- Paul Martin, 21st prime minister of Canada
- Alan Alda, American actor
- David Sanborn, American saxophonist
- Dinah Shore, American actress/singer
- Frida Kahlo, Mexican painter
- Judy Collins, American singer/songwriter

Clearly, these people suffered to varying degrees, with many of them like Jack Nicklaus experiencing mild cases and all of them going on to lead productive lives. Judy Collins spent a couple of months in a hospital in isolation when she was eleven (1950). Alan Alda contracted the disease when he was seven years old (1943) and was subsequently subjected to extremely painful treatments. Fortunately, the treatments helped a great deal and he was able to regain movement.[16] Probably everyone who has studied any American history knows that FDR's dedication to helping people with polio, including himself, led to his founding of a rehabilitation organization in Warm Springs, Georgia. The result was the first hospital (and for many years, the only one) that was devoted exclusively to the treatment of polio victims. That organization became the National Foundation for Infantile Paralysis; we know it as the March of Dimes, which funded the research for vaccines developed by Jonas Salk and Albert Sabin. With the introduction of their vaccines, polio eventually became part of America's past instead of its present. We do, however, have people like many of those just mentioned who are still here to remind us of polio's horrors.

Polio can cause acute paralysis and often permanent physical disability and death. Many children were left in braces, on crutches or in wheelchairs for the rest of their lives. Comparatively speaking, Judy Collins and Alan Alda were lucky; FDR was one of those who was visibly crippled for the remainder of his life. They were far more fortunate than the character portrayed in the 2012 movie, *The Sessions*, in which a poet paralyzed by polio spends his time in an iron lung, a chamber enabling someone to breathe after loss of the muscle control needed to do it independently.

The inactivated polio vaccine (IPV) is the formula currently given to patients. In 1988, the IPV replaced the oral polio vaccine previously used. Baby boomers can still remember lining up at school for sugar cubes infused with this early vaccine. (Currently, oral polio vaccine is still available and used in countries where there is wild polio—meaning it's endemic to the area—because it gives more gastrointestinal immunity while the IPV more specifically protects the nervous system.)

Before this vaccine was available in the 1950s, about 20,000 cases of polio were reported each year in the United States and about 350,000 cases were reported worldwide. By starting vaccination in the United States in 1955, we saw a drop to only ten cases by 1979 and then watched that total eventually move down to zero. Side effects with the IPV are usually just mild soreness at the injection site.

The oral polio vaccine did have a very rare incidence of vaccine-induced polio, with a reported rate of about one in 2.4 million people. These cases typically occurred in adults receiving the vaccine and almost none were in the United States. Compare those numbers to the potential rate of infection of one in 11,000 that we could have seen in 1988 if there were no vaccine program. That one in 11,000 number is based on the population of 226 million Americans at that time and 20,000 cases annually. So even though oral polio vaccine was known to cause this issue, it was much better than the alternative without it.

However, the medical community was not happy with *anyone* having polio, so the United States turned to the IPV in 1988 and since then we haven't seen any of those vaccine-induced cases. The World Health Assembly, which is the decision-making body of the World Health Organization, also agreed unanimously in 1988 to eradicate polio from the globe. Since then, rates have plummeted to only 2,000 cases in 2006 and 1,600 cases in 2007. In 2010 there were just 540 cases globally. The official statistic from WHO is that polio cases have decreased by over 99 percent since the 1988 commitment to eliminate it.[17]

There is an interesting footnote to the "vaccine-induced polio" problem. When the cases were studied, it was ultimately determined that the real culprit was probably an immune deficiency the individual had, known as X-linked agammaglobulinemia. This is a rare immune deficiency that doesn't allow a person to make any antibody in the body; therefore, the person cannot react to an illness or vaccine correctly.

ROTAVIRUS VACCINE

Rotavirus is the number one reason for hospitalization admissions of children due to gastroenteritis in the United States. That means it sends about three million kids to the doctor and 55,000 to the hospital every year with dehydrating diarrhea. Adults who have a rotavirus infection may experience few or no symptoms, but young children tend to have fever, nausea, vomiting, cramps and watery diarrhea. They might also have a persistent cough and runny nose. It's very contagious, so if one child at daycare has it, it can easily spread to all the other children.

If all people, including children, washed their hands throughout the day as though they were about to perform surgery, it would be easy to stop the spread of rotavirus. But most people don't, so the rotavirus vaccine is given to mitigate the risks of catching it.

The rotavirus vaccine generally used is either RotaTeq (Merck) or Rotarix (GlaxoSmithKline). The vaccine covers five serotypes/subtypes of the rotavirus, which are the ones that typically cause disease. Vaccinations have resulted in a reduction of rotavirus-related hospitalizations and doctor visits. In the studies leading up to the FDA's approval of RotaTeq, the vaccine prevented 74 percent of all rotavirus gastroenteritis cases and 98 percent of the severe cases for the nearly 7,000 infants from the United States and Finland who participated. In addition, RotaTeq reduced hospitalization for gastroenteritis due to rotavirus by 96 percent through two years of age.[18]

A previous rotavirus vaccine called RotaShield (Wyeth), which was a series of three injections, stayed on the market only nine months before being withdrawn in 1999. It didn't take long for case reports of *intussusception* (a type of bowel obstruction) to emerge after the vaccine first started being administered. After the vaccine was withdrawn, studies concluded the vaccine wasn't the cause of the intussusceptions; it was the schedule for giving it. Research deemed the situation a "temporal association with intussesception events that occurred in vaccinated infants," however, RotaShield remained doomed.[19] The actual incidence of intussusception turned out to be 1.5 to four cases per 1,000 live births, with a peak age range of nine to twenty-four months.

In the gap between RotaShield being taken off the market and when RotaTeq was released and recommended for worldwide vaccination, about five million children died of dehydration from rotavirus (about 1,600 children daily under five years of age).

Even on his modified schedule of vaccinations, Robert Sears concurs with the AAP that the rotavirus vaccine should be given at two months.

VACCINES AT FOUR MONTHS
Vaccines given at the four-month visit are the same vaccines as those given at two months. This is done to kick the immunity back up and keep the body "interested" in fighting the targeted diseases. Babies are at some of the highest risks for the targeted conditions.

VACCINES AT SIX MONTHS
Vaccines given at the six-month visit are the same vaccines as those given at two and four months. But now there's one more: At six months, influenza vaccine is added to the mix. Typically, the process involves one shot at six months and then a repeat flu vaccine thirty days after the first vaccination to complete the immunity. After that, they just need one flu vaccine annually. (The discussion of influenza and the influenza vaccine is primarily in chapter 4.)

Important health issues start emerging at about four to six months of age. Ear infections and other illnesses start occurring as the maternal antibodies inside the baby go away after delivery. The intent is that vaccines such as Prevnar (pneumococcal vaccine) help reduce the number of ear infections caused by the subtypes in the vaccine.

Here's a fact that many anti-vaccination mothers use in their defense: There are lower rates of ear infections in kids who are breastfeeding. The reason for this is that these babies are continually getting extra antibodies from their mothers' breast milk. Formula-fed kids are lacking in this extra immunity. It should be noted, however, that while these advantages provided by breastfeeding are long-lasting, they don't last forever. Most pediatricians would agree it's a good idea to keep breastfeeding *and* vaccinate. This topic gets more in-depth coverage in chapter 7.

VACCINES AT NINE MONTHS

At nine months, there are typically no shots at the well visit unless you are behind. Depending on the season, however, the doctor may suggest a flu vaccine.

There has been recent research related to vaccines for meningococcal disease that would enable vaccination to begin at nine months and eventually maybe even younger. Right now, the current Menactra vaccine has indications for more routine use on children that young if the appropriate clinical situation exists. Menactra is manufactured by Sanofi Pasteur, which now states in its literature that the vaccine is "given to people nine months through fifty-five years of age to help prevent meningococcal disease (including meningitis)."[20] They can state this, because in April of 2011 the FDA approved the vaccine's use for children down to nine months of age with a booster recommended at twelve months.

Meningococcal disease is not one of those that moves slowly enough to let the immune system summon the right antibodies to the front line and create a strong defense. An infected body can die within hours.

VACCINES AT TWELVE TO FIFTEEN MONTHS

As the AAP chart indicates, the third dose of Hep B vaccine might be given at any point within the six-month to fifteen-month time-frame, so this isn't as rigid as some critics of the schedule suggest. At fifteen months, there's the fourth and final dose of DTaP. At twelve to fifteen months, it's the next dose of Hib vaccine and Pneumoccal conjugate, brand name Prevnar 13. And as with the Hep B vaccine, the final dose of IPV vaccine for polio might be given any time between six months and fifteen months. Other than that, we're talking about a seasonal flu shot and the one that has probably caused the most controversy of all: MMR.

The measles/mumps/rubella (MMR) vaccine given at twelve to fifteen months is the one targeted by many concerned parents as being linked to the onset of autism. While the discussion of MMR vaccine and autism receives in-depth attention in chapter 5, it should be stated here that children with autism spectrum disorder (ASD) usually show signs in the first year.[21]

The dangers of measles, mumps and rubella, as well as the rise in rates of occurrence since more parents started questioning vaccine safety, were covered in chapter 1. Here, it is important to note that parents are challenged with making a decision about administering this vaccine at a time when a great many changes are going on with their baby. It may also be a time when they are thrilled at how the child is thriving—walking, communicating, socializing. It is no wonder that suspicions about what's best for the emerging toddler would come into play and a key suspicion relates to the value and safety of the MMR vaccine.

The final two vaccines in the line-up for children in the twelve-to-fifteen-month age range are varicella and hepatitis A. The varicella vaccine protects against chickenpox, which is often dismissed as one of those childhood diseases that is annoying, but not serious. However, the disease can still kill; the people who are most vulnerable to serious effects of chickenpox are infants and adults. We've spoken with adults who remember chickenpox parties in pre-vaccine days, that is, pre-1995: After one kid got it, rather than wait for it to circulate in school, the parents simply put the kids in the same room and let them all catch it. The short-term result was an itchy, ugly, blister-like rash; the long-term result was lifelong immunity. Even though most school-age kids may be able to handle the effects of varicalla-zoster virus, if their unvaccinated baby brother or sister gets it, the virus could be life-threatening—as the roughly 100 deaths per year and 11,000 hospitalizations that occurred in pre-vaccine days illustrate.

Like hepatitis B, hepatitis A is a liver infection, but it's contracted in a different way. The usual way to get it is from fecal matter. You could touch an object or ingest food or drink that's been contaminated and even a microscopic amount of fecal matter from an infected person sends that disease straight to you. Knowing this, you may no longer think it's strange that some people will not touch the door handle of a bathroom with their bare hands! Knowing this, you may also see why a toddler is particularly vulnerable. Touching everything and everyone as he makes his way from chair to table to television set to floor, if there's an infected person in the house, he's at risk. Unfortunately, many people who are infected don't know it, so they feel fine themselves but unwittingly spread the disease and make others sick.

The Hep A vaccine was licensed the same year as the chickenpox vaccine—1995—and typically the side effect is soreness at the injection site.

ARGUMENTS TO PULL BACK FROM THE SCHEDULE

Every vaccine mentioned by brand name comes with a warning from the manufacturer.

In this chapter alone, we have referenced several different vaccines commonly administered to babies: Hep B, DTaP, Hib, pneumococcal disease, IPV, rotavirus, MMR, varicella and Hep A. Descriptions of safety information and potential side effects accompany all of these vaccines and can be found online.

The information on safety and side effects is there for legal reasons as well as health reasons: This *could* happen; that *might* happen if you have a certain pre-existing condition; on rare occasions, something else *could* happen. They mention even the most remote and extreme side effects possible, because they have to disclose every one they've identified.

Coauthor Maryann has a story from her own life that captures "every mother's nightmare" as it might pertain to side effects from a vaccine. Flagyl, which is a version of metronidazole, is often given to counter protozoal infections like giardia. Maryann happened to pick up the giardia parasite by accidentally ingesting contaminated water; she started her course of Flagyl immediately after diagnosis. She drank no alcohol during the time she was taking Flagyl—an essential step in averting some very unpleasant side effects. After a day of taking the medication, she started having some noticeable, but relatively mild, reactions. Then she developed a rash. She looked at the product literature and started mentally checking off all of the other side effects that she'd seemed to be having. On day five, she was rushed to the emergency room of the hospital, because she could hardly breathe. It was one of those extreme, rare side effects.

Put yourself in a mother's shoes who has experienced something like Maryann's encounter with Flagyl—that "anything can happen" feeling. Naturally, you don't want anything bad to happen to your baby. So imagine your two-month old is scheduled to receive a dose of rotavirus vaccine tomorrow. You go online and download the patient information on the product your doctor said she's using: RotaTeq. Written in layman's language, you see a section called "What are the possible side effects of RotaTeq?" You don't like the beginning about possible diarrhea and runny nose, but you can live with it. And then you read on:

Call your child's doctor or go to the emergency department right away if your child has any of the following problems after getting RotaTeq, even if it has been several weeks since the last dose, because these may be signs of a serious problem called intussusception:

- bad vomiting
- bad diarrhea
- severe stomach pain
- blood in the stool.

Intussusception happens when a part of the intestine gets blocked or twisted.

Since FDA approval, reports of infants with intussusception following RotaTeq have been received by the Vaccine Adverse Event Reporting System (VAERS). Intussusception occurred days and sometimes weeks after vaccination. Some infants needed hospitalization, surgery on their intestines or a special enema to treat this problem. Death due to intussusception has occurred.

Other reported side effects include:

+ allergic reactions, which may be severe and may include face and mouth swelling, difficulty breathing, wheezing, hives and/or skin rash.
+ Kawasaki disease (a serious condition that can affect the heart; symptoms may include fever, rash, red eyes, red mouth, swollen glands, swollen hands and feet and if not treated, death can occur).

Call your doctor right away if your child has any side effects that concern you or seem to get worse.

These are NOT all the possible side effects of RotaTeq. You can ask your doctor for a more complete list.[22]

It's one thing to face a list of negative outcomes when you are an adult making a decision for yourself. But when you're a parent and your child is two months old, a list like this could be frightening. Your pediatrician emphasizes the protective benefits of the vaccine and downplays the possibility of a severe side effect occurring, because he or she has ascertained that the benefits far outweigh the risks. Remember that it's your doctor's job to protect your baby, too. But you are haunted by "the list." You go ahead with the dose of RotaTeq, but keep watching your baby for any problem. You become convinced that even the slightest deviation from "normal" is a side effect of the vaccine.

At that point, after one or more vaccines have already been given, some parents decide that they will take measures to ostensibly mitigate the risk or they simply won't take the risk again. They pull back from the schedule, perhaps completely. Many seek alternative schedules based on what they learn from "trusted sources."

In his alternate schedule of vaccinations, Sears gives ten reasons why he recommends spreading out the vaccines in this early period of a child's life. Rather than administering them at two, four, six, twelve and fifteen months as described earlier in this chapter, he calls for immunizations of no more than two vaccines at a time at two, three, four, five, six, seven, nine, twelve, fifteen and eighteen months. One of the reasons centers on side effects. Of his schedule, Sears says, "It gives no more than two vaccines at a time to limit potential side effects. We don't know if giving six simultaneous vaccines causes more side effects, but again, giving fewer is a reasonable precaution."[23]

Similarly, Sears' spread-out schedule reflects his belief that no more than one aluminum-containing vaccine should be given to a child during these early months "so infants can process the aluminum without it reaching toxic levels."[24] (Aluminum's role in vaccines and alleged dangers are discussed in depth in chapter 6.) Some of the other reasons are corollaries to these two having to do with a baby's ability to take in only so much at one time—whether that means chemical additives or live viruses. Others reflect Sears' belief in the relatively low risk of an infant or very young child being exposed to rubella and hepatitis B, for example.

But Sears isn't the only one who proposes an alternative schedule. Another alternative schedule was developed by Stephanie Cave, an MD formerly in family practice and author of *What Your Doctor May Not Tell You About™ Children's Vaccinations.* Her schedule is far more restrictive than Sears', with most visits to the doctor involving only one injection.[25] In addition, she calls for the Hep B vaccine only if the mother is Hep B positive.

Based on a physician's willingness to bend to the will of parents, the potential variations on the schedule are enormous. The title of a *New York Times* article on March 2, 2015, sums up the situation: "Most Doctors Give In to Request by Parents to Alter Vaccine Schedules."[26] It reflects the findings of a survey published that day in the journal *Pediatrics,* which asked 534 primary care physicians how often parents shifted the vaccination schedule for children under the age of two. Of those 534 physicians, 93 percent reported incidences on a regular basis. A third of them said they generally gave in; another third said they sometimes did what the parents wanted.

With statistics like these, one might argue that either doctors also have concerns about the vaccination schedule or they simply don't want to lose patients (that is to say, income), so they accommodate the parents.

ARGUMENTS TO STICK WITH THE SCHEDULE

The vaccination schedule has developed over the past 100 years, with the vaccination for whooping cough entering first in 1914. A sentiment behind the ACIP and AAP schedule of vaccinations might be best summarized by a phrase from Shakespeare's *Henry VI*, Part 1, Act III: "Defer no time, delays have dangerous ends." Translation: "You'll be damned sorry if you procrastinate." That's because, when a child or adult receives a vaccine, it is intimately tied to the time of life and seasonal and other environmental conditions when the threats from vaccine-preventable diseases are greatest or about to be at their greatest.

Vaccines on the schedule for newborns through fifteen months are there because that is when a baby is most susceptible to disease. Doctors are well aware of the fact that infants who have gone full-term tend to have a boost of protection from infectious diseases thanks to the mother and the mother's milk; babies born prematurely don't receive as much protection. Regardless of that probable advantage enjoyed by the full-term, breast-fed infant, the overwhelming majority of the medical community takes a conservative approach to vaccinations, because the consequences of exposing an infant to a serious infectious disease due to delays in vaccination are potentially devastating. It's somewhat analogous to getting the scheduled maintenance done on your car: If you don't, you might be fine or your brakes might fail on the highway. In its briefing for parents on the vaccination schedule, The

Children's Hospital of Philadelphia notes: "If a baby is not too young to get the disease, she is not too young to get the vaccine."[27]

In proposing his alternative vaccine schedule, Sears makes a few arguments that may be true, at least in part, but they are far from the "last word" on risks, benefits and sound parental decision-making. For example, he focuses on parents pushing back and taking control; however, there is a way to do those things that is productive in terms of understanding the risks and benefits of the current schedule. Parents can push back and take control by asking good questions and not stopping until they get good answers. And they need to start with their doctor—the person they selected to help care for the health of their infant. (Exceptions to this are obviously people who don't believe in participating in any mainstream medicine; their situation is discussed later in this book.)

We wouldn't disagree with Sears that many doctors who administer vaccines are not current on the studies and technically that means their knowledge of vaccines would not qualify them as experts. However, unlike the dark days before the World Wide Web, research is now readily accessible and pediatricians and family doctors should be encouraged to access it. In 1993, when coauthor Maryann was researching her first book on medical technology, she went to the National Library of Medicine in Bethesda, Maryland and flashed her "Patron Card" to get copies of studies. Now, doctors are able to access those studies quickly online, as well as read the product information from vaccine manufacturers and put the two together at the request of a concerned parent. The doctor works for you, not the other way around, so don't be afraid to ask questions. For example, a mother who is concerned about side effects of RotaTeq could ask the doctor: "What do the studies say about the possibilities of intussusception occurring?"

PubMed, an online service of the National Library of Medicine, indicates that of the 9,063 studies in its database on intussusception, 2,907 address cases in children and forty-five specifically reference RotaTeq and the issue of the risk of intussusceptions after vaccination.[28] The most current are at the top. The doctor reads a new one called "Intussusception risk after rotavirus vaccination in U.S. infants." In this massive study published in the February 6, 2014, issue of the *New England Journal of Medicine*, the analyses included 507,874 first doses of RotaTeq. The conclusion found it was "associated with approximately 1.5 excess cases of intussusceptions per 100,000 recipients of the first dose."[29] The mother's question is answered with solid data, not a dismissive, "Trust me on this."

In trying to make informed decisions about the vaccine schedule, parents might have concerns about additives as well as side effects. They wonder if Sears is right about aluminum and consider his advice to not give more than one aluminum-containing vaccine at a time in the infant years.

A point about the schedule and individual vaccines which needs to be made emphatically is that any substance can be toxic at the wrong dosage. In April 2015, Lacey Spears was convicted of murdering her five-year-old child by giving him too much salt. She poisoned him with a substance that many of us use every day. It doesn't make sense that it would be the vaccine introducing unsafe levels of aluminum into an infant's system since such miniscule amounts are used—and the schedule reflects the facts that physicians and other scientists took those amounts into consideration. Instead, if there are doubts about the level of aluminum in the infant's system, it would be appropriate to look at what other, more significant sources of aluminum to which the baby is exposed: "[In the first six months] a baby will get 2.5 times the amount of aluminum [in vaccines] from breast milk, ten times the aluminum from infant formula and thirty times the aluminum from soy-based formula."[30] To clarify the numbers used, this is based on a baby getting about four milligrams from vaccines in the first six months of life if all the vaccines on the schedule are administered and in the same period getting ten milligrams from breast milk, forty milligrams from formula and 120 milligrams from soy-based formula.[31]

There are good arguments in favor of revisiting the schedule and good arguments for maintaining it. That's probably the fairest assessment we could make. The strength of science is on the side of maintaining it, but intellectual curiosity to find a "better way" should never be discounted. After all, that curiosity led to the development of the immunization schedule in the first place.

CHAPTER 3

How Do Vaccines Affect Young Children and Adolescents?

Many people in their fifties and sixties today have no recollection of getting vaccines in their teenage years, except for maybe a tetanus shot when they stepped on a rusty nail or they got bitten by the family cat. Adolescents and older teenagers are now very much included in the vaccination schedule of the twenty-first century; there is a series of vaccinations given to them throughout the period of eighteen months to eighteen years.

In this chapter we'll debate the dramatic changes in the immunization schedule since the late twentieth century, including the introduction of a catch-up schedule and the first "teen vaccine"—the human papillomavirus (HPV) vaccine, first licensed in 2006. As a preface to this discussion, we'll look at how the current vaccination schedule took shape and then examine the individual diseases that the vaccines cover in the eighteen-month to eighteen-year age span.

The official vaccination schedule, which is approved by ACIP, AAP and the American Academy of Family Physicians (AAFP), was not adopted until 1995. Prior to that, there was a schedule but it lacked the month-by-month precision that we see on the tables such as those included in this chapter and chapter 2.

In the 1940s, there was a recommendation to get children vaccinated for diphtheria, tetanus and pertussis. A combined vaccine had been developed to get the job done; we still rely on a combination vaccine today (DTaP), which was subsequently combined with others to cover a total of five diseases. A smallpox vaccine was also on the schedule in the 1940s, but was ultimately removed from the list in 1980 when smallpox was considered eradicated globally. By the 1950s, children received the vaccine to prevent polio. The measles, mumps and rubella (MMR) vaccine was added to list for children in the 1970s. By that time, the fifty- and sixty-year-old people of today were in high school, in college and/ or working, so they never got the MMR injection. Many have vivid memories of waking up to grossly swollen glands in the throat area from the mumps and itching all over with a case of the measles. A lot of parents were aware that these diseases were more than an inconvenience—mumps can cause sterility in males and measles can cause inflammation of the brain, for example—but many were *not* aware or never saw a severe response to the diseases, even though "everybody got them."

By the 1970s, many kids were immunized from tetanus, diphtheria, pertussis (whooping cough), polio, measles, mumps and rubella. All seven were covered in three vaccines: polio, DTP and MMR. The list grew as vaccines were developed for more diseases. (Chapter 10, on the future of vaccination, gives a close look at the technologies that evolved over this period and the technologies evolving now that have enabled the development of new vaccines.)

The first *Haemophilus influenza* type b (Hib) vaccine emerged in 1985, but had to go through some refinement before it officially made the list in the late 1980s. *Haemophilus influenza* is a bacterium, but it got its name—and it stuck—in 1892 when Hib was discovered in a group of influenza patients. This was before scientists knew that the flu originated from a virus, so they inferred that Hib was the cause.

A few years later Hep B was added. The process of developing the Hep B vaccine took nearly twenty years, but it took another five years to create one that the medical community and marketplace really embraced. Then it took another decade to get it on the list of scheduled vaccinations. The Hep B that was finally accepted was the first human vaccine produced by recombinant DNA methods, so no human blood products were used in its synthesis.

In 1995, ACIP, AAP and AAFP launched the practice of updating the schedule annually. It was a robust effort involving a lot more information for physicians than had been previously provided automatically. There was detailed information about the vaccines on the list, including specific age- and dosage-related guidelines, as well as a briefing on emerging vaccines as they were added to the schedule.[1]

Since that first list, which contained nine recommended vaccines, many others have been added:

- Varicella (chickenpox) vaccine was added in 1995, with a booster added in 2006.
- Hepatitis A vaccine was added about the same time.
- Rotavirus vaccine had its ups and downs shortly after introduction in 1999, but following refinements by more than one company, it was deemed safe and effective and then fully endorsed by 2009.
- Pneumococcal vaccine first started being recommended in 2000, but it wasn't until 2010 that a new formulation (Prevnar 13), considered much more effective, was introduced. Pneumococcal vaccine has an unusually long history of development, with the initial efforts to produce it having occurred in 1911; after that it went through three phases of development over eight decades.[2]

- Influenza vaccine has one of the same "fathers" as polio vaccine—Jonas Salk. He and Thomas Francis formulated the first flu vaccine in 1938 and the first major rounds of patients were US military personnel in World War II. About forty years later, in 1979, the flu vaccine became part of a public vaccination program when there was tremendous fear over an outbreak of swine flu. Finally, in 2012, the AAP recommended annual influenza vaccinations for anyone over six months old.
- Meningococcal vaccine is a late addition to the list, but it has a caveat: It can be given to children as young as nine months when they are considered high risk; other than that, it's part of the schedule for older kids.
- Human papillomavirus (HPV) vaccine was approved in 2006, with pre-adolescent and teenage girls being the first targeted population; the United States officially began including boys in the HPV immunization program in 2011.

There are many other licensed vaccines besides the ones on this list, but they are administered on an as-needed basis as opposed to being part of the schedule. Rabies and yellow fever vaccine are two examples.

The schedule is designed to reflect the needs of the population in general—people of all ages in their normal environments coming into contact with dangerous diseases that are airborne, blood-borne, fluid-borne or somehow transmitted through touch. Communities of all sizes throughout the country have mixed populations because of immigration, migration and travel. And people from communities of all sizes travel to places like Disneyland in California and Central Park in New York to enjoy new experiences. So in addition to the daily environments of schools, grocery stores and walking down the street, all of these occurrences that involve a diversity of people and conditions contribute to what constitutes the "normal environments." Hence, we are working with an immunization schedule that protects against diseases we may rarely see in our hometown, but they still have a profound effect on the health and mortality rates of people from other countries.

VACCINES AT EIGHTEEN TO TWENTY-THREE MONTHS

If the child has not received a third dose of the Hep B and polio vaccine, this marks the end of the timeframe in which these vaccines are given to have the desired impact (from six months to eighteen months). Similarly, the window for the fourth dose of DTaP is fifteen to eighteen months. With the Hep A vaccine, the recommended time for the two-dose series is anywhere from nine months to twenty-three months.

There is also the annual influenza vaccination, the administration of which is typically tied to the flu season; so the first one might be given at six months at the earliest or it might be given several months later. When you look at these vaccination schedules, you might find the reference to "one or two doses" to be confusing. Which is it—one or two? Children receiving the flu vaccine for the first time typically get two doses, which are given at least twenty-eight days apart. This is a determination with which your doctor can help you; there is some wiggle room on this depending on risk factors in the environment and the child's overall health.

VACCINES AT TWO TO THREE YEARS

The one vaccine you see on the schedule in this time period is for the flu. Since flu season is annual, the vaccination is annual. When a child becomes two years old, some of the cautions about flu vaccine come into play. Along with the cautions come options. In other words, flu vaccines are essentially created equal, but they don't perform identically, so you have choices to make with your children. This is one of those many situations where doing some homework and having an actual conversation with your child's doctor makes sense.

EIGHTEEN MONTHS TO EIGHTEEN YEARS

VACCINES	18 MOS	19–23 MOS	2–3 YRS	4–6 YRS	7–8 YRS	9–10 YRS	11–12 YRS	13–15 YRS	16–18 YRS
Hepatitis B (Hep B)	←3rd dose→								
Diphtheria, tetanus and acellular pertussis (DTaP: <7 yrs)	←4th dose→			←5th dose→					
Tetanus, diphtheria and acellular pertussis (Tdap: ≥7 yrs)							(Tdap)		
Inactivated poliovirus (IPV) (<18 yrs)	←3rd dose→			←4th dose→					
Influenza (IIV; LAIV) 2 doses for some	Annual vaccination (IIV only) 1 or 2 doses	Annual vaccination (LAIV or IIV) 1 or 2 doses				Annual vaccination (LAIV or IIV) 1 dose only			
Measles, mumps, rubella (MMR)				←2nd dose→					
Varicella (VAR)				←2nd dose→					
Hepatitis A (Hep A)	←2 dose series→								
Human papillomavirus (HPV2: females only; HPV4: males and females)							←3 dose series→		
Meningococcal (Hib-Men-CY ≥ 6 weeks; MenACWY-D ≥9 mos; MenACWY-CRM ≥ 2 mos)							←1st dose→		Booster

There are two different kinds of flu vaccine: inactivated influenza vaccine (IIV) and live, attenuated influenza vaccine (LAIV). They are administered in two different ways: IIV is given by injection and LAIV is given in the form of a nasal spray. Although either can be given—and IIV is often the one that's readily available—LAIV is preferred by many parents, because it doesn't involve a shot. The added benefit to LAIV is that it seems to be far more effective with young children. In fact, the CDC says that the nasal spray prevented about 50 percent more cases of flu than the flu shot in younger children. For this reason, the CDC now recommends the LAIV nasal spray for healthy children between the ages of two and eight years old whenever it's available.[3]

Notice the qualifying word "healthy." There are certain types of children for whom LAIV is considered a bad choice. It's recommended that the following receive a flu shot instead:

- Children (or people of any age) who have previously experienced severe allergic reactions to LAIV, any of its components or any other influenza vaccine[4]
  - o In addition to the active ingredients in the vaccine that are a source of immunity, the inactive ingredients in the nasal spray (known as FluMist in the United States and Canada and manufactured by MedImmune) are ethylene diaminetetraaceticacid (EDTA), monosodium glutamate, hydrolyzed porcine gelatin, arginine, sucrose, dibasic potassium phosphate, monobasic potassium phosphate, gentamicin sulfate and egg protein.[5]
  - o Based on the list of ingredients, children with a history of egg allergy need to stay away from the nasal spray.
- Children who regularly take medicines containing aspirin
- Children from ages two to four who have had asthma or wheezing during the previous twelve months

- Children who have taken influenza antiviral medications such as Tamiflu® or Relenza® within the previous forty-eight hours
- Children who have a weakened immune system—that is, immunosuppressed children
  - o Immunosuppression can describe the condition that occurs when a person is fighting a chronic illness. It can also be induced for some medical reason. Cortisone is an example of a substance deliberately used to suppress the immune system.

The CDC also points out that there currently isn't enough data about the effect of the nasal spray on kids with health conditions that put them at increased risk of serious flu complications, such as diabetes, heart disease and neurological conditions.[6]

Some of the side effects of flu vaccine, no matter what kind the child gets, look like flu symptoms: runny nose, headache, wheezing, vomiting, muscle aches and fever. The big difference to watch out for is the duration and intensity. Side effects of the vaccine usually don't last long and they are milder than actual flu symptoms.

VACCINES AT FOUR TO SIX YEARS

Much of the anecdotal "evidence" online about children having adverse reactions to vaccines seems centered on this age group. There are frightening stories of seizures and black-outs after any one or all of the vaccines recommended from ages four to six, namely the fifth dose of DTaP, fourth dose of polio, second dose of MMR and second dose of varicella (chickenpox).

One mother, who conveyed having a PhD in chemistry, described a heart-stopping experience involving her four-year-old daughter. The pre-schooler had just received the DTaP and varicella vaccines in addition to a capillary blood draw:

> Immediately after the injections, as the nurse was returning the syringes to her little tray, my daughter, still sitting on my

lap, thrashed—her arm narrowly missing my head—then her eyes rolled back and she became unconscious. I managed to lay her down on the bench without dropping her and the nurse brought the pediatrician back into the room. A few moments later, my daughter came to, finding both her doctor and her mom hovering over her.[7]

This story comes from an informed mother who said she had read the Vaccination Information Sheets provided by her doctor. She was aware of the one in 14,000 chance of a child having a seizure after the DTaP vaccination. Based on what happened, how could she not question the safety of the vaccine for her child now? How could she not question the safety of the year-four vaccines for her son, who would be at that age shortly? After all, she reasoned, if there was a genetic component to the reaction, he might have it too. Fortunately, after the initial incident and the various tests that followed, the little girl showed no further signs of problems.

Despite this experience and her consideration of the risks posed to her son, this mother still chose to have him vaccinated when he turned four. She decided that she would rather risk seizure than pertussis, the "hundred day cough."

Her story generated a number of comments online, including a simple question of how someone could remain supportive of vaccinations for her children after going through something like that. In this discussion, an important fact came to light: namely, that the immediacy of the response suggested that whatever was in the needle hadn't even entered the bloodstream yet. A biological response to the vaccine would have taken a little more time.

So what do the medical professionals believe happened? It's something called *vasovagal syncope* and apparently not uncommon immediately after getting a vaccination, although there aren't any published percentages on the rate of occurrence. Here is the CDC's explanation of the phenomenon:

Syncope, also called fainting, is a temporary loss of consciousness as a result of decreased blood flow to the brain. The most common form of fainting is called "vasovagal" fainting. This type of fainting can be triggered by an event associated with pain or anxiety. Some people may experience jerking movements after fainting which are not seizures.[8]

In addition to the emotional stories of parents watching a child faint and/or thrash, probably the most common horror story about the vaccines at ages four to six involves MMR—the vaccine many parents blame for the onset of autism in their child. (An in-depth discussion of the alleged link between MMR and autism is the debate featured in chapter 5 and also covered in chapter 6.)

VACCINES AT SEVEN TO TEN YEARS

This is a "quiet period" in terms of vaccinations, with nothing more on the schedule than the annual flu vaccine. The only exception is if the child gets exposed to a few surprises in terms of the environment; this is a time when parents are more inclined to let their growing children go on wilderness adventures or take trips with the families of friends. At this point, it's not a period of adhering to a vaccination schedule, but rather looking for what different health challenges might be confronting the child because of exposure to new people and new situations.

VACCINES AT ELEVEN TO TWELVE YEARS

About one hundred years before a vaccine was developed to prevent human papillomaviruses (HPV), the medical community suspected an association between cervical cancer and sexual behavior. But those suspicions led to hypotheses that cervical cancer was perhaps a disease resulting from "too many" sexual partners or becoming sexually active at a young age. These are risk factors, just as smoking is a risk factor, but it wasn't until the work of German scientist Harald zur Hausen of the University of Dusseldorf that it became clear what exactly caused nearly all cases of cervical cancer: HPV.

Zur Hausen's search for answers about HPV began in 1979. Within two years, his work yielded astonishing results positively linking HPV to cervical cancer. He contacted pharmaceutical companies about developing an HPV vaccine, but there was no interest "in view of a market analysis conducted by one of [the companies] which indicated that there would be no market available."[9] (Yes, critics of Big Pharma, this is support for your assertion that pharmaceutical companies want to make money. But that doesn't make them inherently evil, careless or exploitive; it makes them businesses.)

Finally, in 2008, two years after an HPV vaccine was added to the list of recommended immunizations beginning in the eleventh or twelfth year, zur Hausen won the Nobel Prize in Medicine, which he shared with two French scientists who were pioneers in AIDS research. The press release announcing his award unequivocally stated the link between his work and saving the lives of countless women:

> Harald zur Hausen was awarded the other half of the Nobel Prize for work which proved that oncogenic human papillomavirus (HPV) caused cervical cancer, the second most common cancer in women. This discovery led to understanding the basis for HPV infection and HPV-induced cancers and the subsequent development of prophylactic vaccines against HPV.[10]

Oncogenic means that it caused tumors, so the reference here is to cancer-causing HPV; there are more than 100 HPV types and some cause low-grade abnormalities, whereas others are the types detected in 99 percent of cervical cancers.[11]

Most people with HPV show no signs of infection. Those who do might have genital warts, recurrent respiratory problems, precursors to cervical cancer or cancer itself. The cancer from HPV isn't necessarily restricted to cervical cancer, either. It can also be anal, vaginal, vulvar, penile or head and neck cancer.

There's no treatment for HPV infection. Rather, the doctor treats the symptoms—warts, abnormal cells in the cervix and so on. This is a compelling reason why the medical community got behind the vaccine: An effective vaccine is a much simpler and far less expensive way to manage the threat of HPV than treating the manifestations of HPV infection.

The resistance coming from some parents relates to how HPV is transmitted: sexual contact. These parents don't want their eleven- and twelve-year-olds given a vaccine that they theoretically shouldn't need if they are behaving themselves. The problem is that sexual intercourse isn't the only type of sexual contact, so kids experimenting with nonpenetrative sexual activity are at risk, too.

In addition to the three-dose series of HPV vaccinations, children in this age group also get their first dose of meningococcal vaccine (Menactra) if they didn't receive it earlier due to being in a high-risk group.

Robert Sears' alternative schedule also calls for both the HPV and meningococcal vaccines in roughly this same time period. He actually puts the ages at twelve and thirteen, instead of eleven and twelve, for the series of three HPV shots and, with the final HPV shot, the meningococcal vaccination.

VACCINES AT THIRTEEN TO EIGHTEEN YEARS
The meningococcal booster and annual flu vaccine are the only ones on the schedule in this age range.

THE CATCH-UP SCHEDULE
There's an easy way and a hard way to grasp the vaccination catch-up schedule. Let's look briefly at the hard way first—the way that doctors need to comprehend it.

The catch-up schedule focuses on the minimum intervals between doses while accounting for the age of the child. It's designed to be used in conjunction with the two tables previously provided in this book. There is no practical reason to insert the catch-up table here, because it's designed for clinicians and contains a lot of "if-then" instructions (you can easily access it on the AAP website). A parent who changed her mind about vaccinating her child and looked into the catch-up schedule would likely be amazed at the level of precision the guidance reflects—frequently noting that there are differences in the intervals depending on what brand of vaccine was given previously.

Here is an example of how specific these catch-up instructions are: If the child didn't start receiving the first of three doses of Hib vaccine at two months, the catch-up schedule calls for a minimum interval of "four weeks if current age is younger than twelve months **and** first dose was administered at younger than age seven months **and** at least one previous dose was PRP-T (ActHib, Pentacel) or unknown." [12] Throughout the instructions, as the quote here suggests, the words "and" and "or" are boldfaced and/or capitalized to call attention to the conditions of the schedule. The instructions after that initial note on "four weeks" go on at length, next clarifying that the minimum interval is as follows:

Eight weeks *and* age twelve through fifty-nine months (as final dose)

- If current age is younger than twelve months **and** first dose was administered at age seven through eleven months; **OR**
- If current age is twelve through fifty-nine months **and** first dose was administered before the first birthday **and** second dose was administered at younger than fifteen months; **OR**

> ✦ If both doses were PRP-OMP (PedvaxHIB; Comvax)
> **and** were administered before the first birthday.

No further doses needed if previous dose was administered at
age fifteen months or older.[13]

A lengthy footnote also accompanies the just cited "abbreviated"
instructions.

Now for the easier way to figure out what the catch-up schedule
is for your children. There is a tool called "Catch-Up Immunization
Scheduler," which was designed in collaboration with the CDC and
different departments at Georgia Tech University. Using this tool,
parents enter their child's birth date and vaccination history to
generate a customized catch-up schedule.[14]

So if you want to know when to coordinate times with your
doctor for catch-up vaccinations, use the scheduling software. If
you want to know why the software gave you the answers it did,
then read the full set of instructions on the AAP website.

CHALLENGING THE CURRENT VACCINATION SCHEDULE

Now that it's easy to go online and access the product safety information associated with every vaccine that could potentially be
given to a child, it seems logical that certain types of individuals
would do it—and allow what they learn to influence their decision
whether to vaccinate and/or when to vaccinate. Those types of
individuals could include:

- Intellectually curious people who trust their knowledge and
  inductive reasoning skills
- People who are looking for science-based reasons to get an exemption from the vaccination schedule
- Parents with a family history of unusual or extreme responses
  to medicines and/or food and/or environmental factors

Each type could potentially offer challenges to the current vaccination schedule. The question is: Is "their" science better than the science behind the current schedule of the ACIP and endorsed by the AAP and AAFP?

Earlier in this chapter, we told the story of a PhD chemist who chose to continue the vaccination program for her children despite an adverse event. One of the online responses to the experience she shared serves as an enlightening challenge to the current vaccination schedule—it begs for greater consideration of unique health conditions in determining who is vaccinated and when:

> My daughter has Common Variable Immunodeficiency. Her immune system cannot produce adequate antibodies. She now receives antibody replacement, IVIG, every four weeks to protect her from viruses and infections. The CVID wasn't yet diagnosed when she received the MMR and Varicella vaccines. Twenty days later, she had a bulls-eye rash, high fever [and] seizures, followed by regression...She also would regress when she had other febrile events, including after mono and rotovirus. Since she began IVIG twenty-eight months ago, she has not suffered a single febrile event.
>
> She also has a permanent medical exemption to all further vaccination. She hasn't been able to receive a vaccine since she was twenty months old.
>
> CVID is listed as a contraindicated condition to both the MMR and Varicella vaccines.
>
> While I understand my daughter had a reaction due to her rare condition, I honestly don't agree with today's vaccination schedule. Until we can improve upon identifying children with contraindicated conditions, I don't think we should be adding more vaccines...However, you will not catch me blathering on about toxins or aborted fetuses. I cringe whenever I hear anti-vax propaganda. My daughter had a reaction because

she couldn't create antibodies and the virus over-replicated. A wild case of measles or varicella can cause further regression, if not kill her.

I would like to punch the next person squarely in the nose who says "MY unvaccinated child is not a risk to your vaccinated child." Yes, they are very much a risk.[15]

The central message of this mother's post is a call for customization of the vaccine schedule based on her daughter's special condition. But it's normal for any parent to think: *My kid is special. There's no kid quite like mine.* From extreme cases such as this one involving CVID, to a more common case of a child being born by Cesarean section versus vaginal birth, the circumstances of gestation and birth along with the issues of genetics and environment make each child "special."

But how could something like a C-section delivery make a difference to your child in relation to infections and perhaps even vaccines? In *Infectious Behavior: Brain-Immune Connections in Autism, Schizophrenia, and Depression*, developmental neurobiologist Paul Patterson notes the potential impact a C-section birth can have on the child:

> The bacteria initially present in the human GI tract come from the mother at birth. The fetus itself is sterile, but a normal vaginal birth coats the newborn with microbes from the mother's birth canal. And in fact, it has recently been reported that babies born by Cesarean section are coated with microbes typically found on the skin of adults. These presumably come from the handling the newborns receive after birth. The effects of such abnormal bacterial colonization on both GI and immune status are largely unknown at present, but studies have indeed linked Cesarean births to increased asthma and allergies in those children. This may be another reason to worry about the very high rates of Cesarean section births in the United States.[16]

But does the reality of child-to-child differences, some of which are subtle and some of which are extreme, contain the substance of a real challenge to the current vaccination schedule? In theory, maybe: If we can have customized shirts, handbags and jeans, why not push for customized vaccination schedules reflecting everything that's known about a child's health history and environment? In reality, however, we all know that makes no sense when you're talking about seventy-three million children under the age of eighteen in the United States alone.[17] We just aren't there yet.

APPRECIATING THE CURRENT VACCINE SCHEDULE

Many who challenge the current vaccination schedule point to the number of vaccines added to the list since the 1980s. They assert it just isn't logical that tiny human beings could handle so much more "stuff" in their developing systems. But the truth is that today's children aren't actually handling as much "stuff" in many cases:

> Indeed, children receive many more vaccines than they did a few decades ago. But years ago vaccines contained many more antigenic components than they do today. Examples of these older immunizations include the smallpox vaccine (no longer administered since smallpox was eliminated from the world through vaccination) that contained thousands of components and the old pertussis vaccine that contained more than 3,000 antigen components; today's pertussis vaccine contains up to five such antigens. A fully immunized two-year-old gets only about 315 components that stimulate the immune system.[18]

A challenger of the schedule would probably see this data and suggest that, along with more vaccines, children receive a lot more inactive ingredients, too. Known as *excipients*, these inactive ingredients are a main target of criticism from people such as Robert Sears. (Excipients receive in-depth focus in chapter 6.)

It's important to note in a discussion on the value of the vaccine schedule that Sears identifies as pro-vaccine. He just doesn't agree that the immunizations need to occur when currently prescribed and he disagrees about the necessity of some of them at any time. The counter to his alternative schedule relates specifically to what the mainstream medical community (as primarily embodied by the CDC) has determined to be the most ideal program to protect children at the right time and with the right amount of antigens.

We are ending the debate in this chapter with a different reason why people might appreciate the current vaccination schedule: It's about money. In a paper called "Economic Evaluation of the 7-Vaccine Route Children Immunization Schedule in the United States 2001," the authors, with distinguished positions at The United Nations Children's Fund (UNICEF) and the CDC, said this:

> Routine childhood immunization with the seven vaccines was cost saving from the direct cost and societal perspectives, with net savings of $9.9 billion and $43.3 billion, respectively. Without routine vaccination, direct and societal costs of diphtheria, tetanus, pertussis, H influenzae type b, poliomyelitis, measles, mumps, rubella, congenital rubella syndrome, hepatitis B and varicella would be $12.3 billion and $46.6 billion, respectively. Direct and societal costs for the vaccination program were an estimated $2.3 billion and $2.8 billion, respectively. Direct and societal benefit-cost ratios for routine childhood vaccination were 5.3 and 16.5, respectively.[19]

The scientific data cited in other parts of this book have indicated that the current vaccination schedule affords society some tremendous benefits. We are not saying that the schedule is perfect. No one is saying that. Both sides would agree that each child is special.

CHAPTER 4

How Do Vaccines Affect Adults of Any Age?

The main focus of this book is how to best serve the health needs of our children with regards to vaccines. So why do we need a chapter on adults? The answer to this question is two-fold: It involves the attitudes of adults toward vaccination and the reality of adults and children interacting in ways that can transmit disease.

The latter issue has to do with the precautions that are taken (or lack thereof) so adults and children don't "contaminate" each other. In some cases, adults may choose to receive vaccinations that they don't even want their children to get, like the flu vaccine, because they don't want to risk infecting them. The issue of attitudes is more complicated. Attitudes are shaped in many ways: personal experience, imagination, insights from trusted sources, opinions from celebrities, misinformation and other factors that affect our emotions and perception of "truth."

Essayist Eula Biss had an experience that led to an interesting journey toward her own personal "truth" about vaccination. It all began with her pregnancy and asking a few questions about what was best for her son. That, in turn, fueled more questions and led to growing uncertainty about her overall attitude toward vaccines and the immunization program in the United States. Biss ended up writing a book of essays called *On Immunity: An Inoculation*, a 2014 bestseller that reflects a thoughtful exploration of vaccination in relation to culture, race, privilege, medicine, environmentalism, citizenship, government and more. Her book also provides some keen insights into the history of the anti-vaccination movement as well.

Another person taking the same intellectual and emotional journey as Biss could arrive at an entirely different attitude from hers. Starting with the same questions, the two could easily end up on opposite sides of the debate—and that's because it isn't just about information. Each person's "truth" isn't just about facts. Woven into it are all those other factors that affect how we read, how we hear, how we understand and how we process.

ADULT VACCINATION: THE DEBATE BECOMES INTERNAL

Unlike other debate sections in this book, where the points of view of those who have issues with vaccines are contrasted with those of pro-vaccine people, this chapter deals with the formation of attitudes toward vaccination and how different people act on those attitudes. You might think of this debate as the one that goes on inside the mind of an individual person, rather than the one he or she has with someone else.

The centerpiece of the debate is adult flu vaccinations. Some people, without hesitation, say "I get the flu shot every year." Others take different positions at different times: "I never used to get vaccinated, because I thought it wasn't necessary. Then, one year I got really sick, so now I always get it." Still others say they've done it, but "It made me sick so I'll never do it again." Finally, there are people who just plain avoid it. They either never believed it was a good idea or they no longer believe it's a good idea. A subset of the last opinion is that "It doesn't work."

However, attitudes can change. An eighteen-year-old who's convinced she can curb the virus by staying healthy may have a conflicting internal message ten years later when she has a newborn baby to protect. A father of young kids who had superior health for thirty years and thought all vaccines were snake oil might wrestle with that belief when he finds out his own immune system is compromised through a disease like cancer. Each of them not only affects the attitudes of other people, but also has a decision-making role when it comes to vaccinating children. Their internal dialogues are key parts of the vaccination debate.

Vaccination rates are a good starting point to examine different attitudes, because the adult rate of vaccinations is far below the rate for children in most locations. Based on flu vaccination rates between 2011 and 2013 for adults aged eighteen to forty-nine, it appears to be common for this group—which includes many adults who contracted measles, mumps and/or chickenpox when they were kids—to avoid the flu vaccine. As for the older population, vaccination rates suggest there is resistance or at least disinterest in the shingles vaccine: Only 3.9 percent of eligible persons got the vaccine during a three-year study period.[1] According to a study produced by seven researchers affiliated with different divisions of the CDC:

> Vaccinations are recommended throughout life to prevent vaccine-preventable diseases and their sequelae. Adult vaccination coverage, however, remains low for most routinely recommended vaccines and well below *Healthy People 2020* targets.[2]

The questions, skepticism and fear that these adults have fuel attitudes and actions of others about recommended vaccinations.

It's those people in the eighteen to forty-nine age range—the sons, daughters and grandchildren of those not getting shingles vaccinations—who are the generations now pulling back from the vaccine schedule and challenging medical practitioners about the safety of vaccines for their children. There is a convergence of logical issues and strong emotions about the immunization program.

Despite seasonal warnings about the dangers of flu, more than 50 percent of the population of people under sixty-five years old seem unconvinced that the information pertains to them. On average, since the year 2000, influenza kills roughly 33,000 people every year.[3] For comparison, 31,000 people die annually from motor vehicle accidents. It's highly likely that the people who avoid flu vaccinations still put their seatbelt on; the fear of the threat feels different. The flu "feels" like an inconvenience; an auto accident is acutely traumatic.

The CDC offers an analysis of flu vaccination coverage in the United States during the 2012–2013 influenza season:

Coverage among adults eighteen years and older increased with increasing age:

- 18–49 years: 31.1 percent
- 50–64 years: 45.1 percent
- ≥65 years: 66.2 percent[4]

One of the things that Eula Biss learned in her research for *On Immunity* is that there were differences of opinion between whites and people of color, specifically African-Americans and Hispanics. Here is the disparity for the adult population in the 2012–2013 flu season (those over eighteen years old):

- White—44.6 percent
- Black—35.6 percent
- Hispanic—33.8 percent

The disparity is even more remarkable when it comes to shingles vaccine: "Vaccine uptake was low (3.9 percent), particularly among black people (0.3 percent) and those with evidence of low income (0.6 percent)."[5]

In an interview with National Public Radio's Audie Cornish, Biss made a sharp point about choice, using the vaccination rates for children of minorities. However, with the shingles study in mind, one could assert that this reasoning might also contribute to minorities' lower adult vaccination rate as well:

> I think I saw it [the way vaccination intersects with class and race] first when I was researching the demographics of who does and doesn't vaccinate, but also who does and doesn't die of vaccine-preventable diseases. One of the statistics that was interesting to me was that there is a group of people who don't vaccinate at all, who tend to be white, middle class, well-educated. And married mothers. And then there's a group of people whose children are under-vaccinated, meaning they haven't received all of their vaccines and that's the people who are more likely to be black, to live below the poverty line, to be a mother who is not married and has recently moved. So these are people who are not vaccinating not because it's a choice or a position they've taken, but because of the circumstances of their lives. This means that this relatively privileged population can end up spreading disease to people who haven't made that choice.[6]

Julia and her husband not only fit Biss' description of parents who choose not to vaccinate, but also illustrate an important point about how attitudes are formed and sustained. Julia is a young healthcare professional who had her first baby in late 2014. She and her husband, Jake, a graduate student, read Robert Sears' *The Vaccine Book* and decided that the risks of vaccination outweighed the benefits for them. It is important to note that Sears is *not* what one would call an anti-vaxxer. He summarizes his opinion in the afterword of his book as follows: "I do think that vaccines are very important, but I wish more attention were given to safety research and the possible problems with vaccines."[7]

But in processing the content of Sears' book and ultimately making a decision based on that information, Julia and Jake were heavily influenced by their surrounding community. When Jake first entered graduate school two years ago, he and Julia moved to a city that holds a great deal of academic activity and a population that's younger than the national average because of its universities and colleges: Boulder, Colorado. In this city of about 100,000 people, the median family income is close to $115,000—more than twice the national average. They charge shoppers ten cents for every plastic bag they use at the grocery store and Ralph Nader won 10 percent of the city's vote when he ran for President as the Green Party candidate in 1996 and 2000. As Biss indicated in her book, she saw environmentalism and attitudes about corporate America as factors that had a role in the development of an anti-vaccination mindset.

Even though she's been working as a healthcare professional since arriving in the city, Julia never had direct exposure to a case of tetanus, whooping cough, measles, mumps, Hib or chickenpox. She's too young—and/or hasn't traveled enough—to have seen a case of diphtheria, polio or smallpox. She doesn't really know if she's ever come in contact with someone who has hepatitis A or B. She *does*, however, know what the flu looks like and feels like. Because of her higher risk of exposure to influenza in a healthcare environment, she does what all of her colleagues do: She gets an annual flu shot.

Herd immunity for several childhood illnesses no longer exists in Julia's new community in Boulder, so chances are good that when her little girl reaches kindergarten age, Julia will finally get a first-hand look at vaccine-preventable diseases. In the Boulder Valley School District, the average of *completely unvaccinated children* is 25.57 percent.[8] Cases of whooping cough reached epidemic levels in 2012 with 170 cases; the rise continued in 2013 with 193 cases confirmed. An article in *The Atlantic* called Boulder "an experiment-oriented city"[9] and summarized why the rejection of childhood vaccinations is not an uncommon household attitude there.

So Julia and Jake aren't vaccinating their baby, because the risks are too great. But Julia will continue to do what many Boulderites do every year: drop by a grocery store, pharmacy, clinic or hospital for a seasonal flu shot. For added protection (or as an alternative), many of them will also go to a special food market to get the ingredients for "nature's flu shot"—garlic, turmeric powder, ginger powder, cayenne pepper, organic pineapple juice and raw honey.

Unfortunately, influenza disease changes and shifts, so there have been some flu pandemics (large outbreaks) against which the available flu vaccine was far less effective than anyone had hoped. In those years, such as the 2004–2005 season, "nature's flu shot" was just about as effective as the vaccine administered. During that season, 65,000 people died from influenza-related illness.

When the right strain of the flu vaccine is utilized, vaccinated people have an improved chance of staying alive, even during an epidemic. When we get it wrong, though, the vaccine is close to meaningless. According to the CDC, the adjusted overall effectiveness rate was a lowly 10 percent for that disastrous flu season. For comparison purposes, here are the rates for the decade beginning with the 2004–2005 season (Note that the CDC chart does not contain data for the 2008–2009 season):

INFLUENZA SEASON[10]	ADJUSTED OVERALL VACCINE EFFECTIVENESS (%)
2004–05	10
2005–06	21
2006–07	52
2007–08	37
2009–10	56
2010–11	60
2011–12	47
2012–13	49
2013–14	51

Exacerbating the negative attitude toward flu shots because they aren't "100 percent effective" are small studies such as one from 2012 called "Increased risk of non-influenza respiratory virus infections associated with receipt of inactivated influenza vaccine," in which the vaccine didn't perform measurably better than the placebo.[11]

Another factor affecting attitudes toward the flu vaccine is the belief and/or fear some people have that it will make them sick. That is completely false. It may make you feel ill for a couple of days, because your immune system is revving up as though you *were* sick, but you do not get sick from the influenza vaccine.

We want to distinguish between what might be perceived as the flu or flu symptoms and what they actually are. Influenza is a respiratory condition. With it may come chills and fever, coughing and sore throat, congestion, body aches, headache and fatigue. It is not a vomiting and diarrhea illness; that's the stomach flu, more correctly called "viral gastroenteritis." The vaccine is for the true flu, so if you get the other illness, don't conclude that the vaccine didn't work.

Also shaping attitudes toward the flu vaccine for many people—and this applies to a widespread concern related to all vaccines—is fear, particularly fear of the unknown.

The H1N1 flu virus, more commonly known as swine flu, made such a big impression that countless news stories covered it week after week in 2009. H1N1 reached pandemic levels that year and people around the world were frantic about getting a vaccine. When a disease is at your doorstep, just as when smallpox was decimating families or polio put many children into iron lungs for the remainder of their lives, people badly want a vaccine.

But just as people facing smallpox or polio had fears about what contents were in the vaccine, the same was true for people when it came to the swine flu. A common perception was that the vaccine was rushed to market to meet an acute need, so it probably hadn't been tested properly. The truth about the H1N1 vaccine is that it was actually old in 2009, rather than new and dramatic.

H1N1 vaccine was made the same way the other flu vaccines are made. Nothing was added: The standard flu virus has H and N components anyway. For the H1N1, the manufacturers just combined the H1 with the N1 components. Both already existed, they just hadn't been paired yet. No new testing needed to be done since there was nothing new going on.

When it became clear there wouldn't be enough doses of H1N1 vaccine available, a couple of companies put out two "experimental" vaccines that really *were* new and different. To receive one of these vaccines, you had to sign a paper stating that you were getting an "experimental" vaccine and that you understood that was what you were getting. Some people were so scared of H1N1 that they got one of those "experimental" vaccines after considering their perceived risk of getting the flu. Desperation won out over fear.

As a footnote to the H1N1 vaccine discussion, as the previous chart indicates, it had one of the highest effectiveness rates of any vaccine administered within the decade 2005–2014. The only season it was higher was the year after—and that vaccine also contained the H1N1 component.

To recap, the internal debate that many adults have about continuing their own vaccination program often centers on:

- The thinking that surrounds them
- Assumptions about their innate ability to fight infection or the belief that they are in a "safe" environment
- The perception that some vaccines don't really work
- The suspicion that vaccines will make them sick
- Fear, usually from being under-informed

When adults have the ability to influence the vaccination program for their children, the attitudes they develop about their own vaccinations can have far-reaching consequences.

FINAL NOTES ON ADULT VACCINES

Earlier in this chapter, we noted that nearly 33,000 people die of the flu every year. The flu can set you up for a secondary bacterial pneumonia, which is one of the ten most deadly diseases. In fact, lower respiratory illnesses are at the very top of the list. Typically, secondary pneumonia with influenza is staphylococcus aureus—staph infection. Almost everybody has heard of an aunt or an uncle who had staph in an elbow or in a foot. It's commonly known that staph infections are grave and they are scary. As of this writing, we have a bacterium called Methicillin-resistant Staphylococcus aureus (MRSA). That means it is resistant to most of the antibiotics which are available to treat it.

Although we have more than 100 different antibiotics to choose from, there are only seven classes among them: penicillins, cephalosporins, macrolides, fluoroquinolones, sulfonamides, tetracyclines and aminoglycosides. A couple of outpatient oral antibiotics are used for treating the conditions related to staph.

Right now, physicians see tons of skin conditions with abscesses from staph. If you get the infection in your blood or your lung, the odds of death are fairly high. There are a few IV treatments that can possibly be used, but they do not guarantee that you are going to survive. By getting a flu vaccine, you can potentially protect yourself from this secondary complication, which is what usually kills most people.

To be specific, it is usually the pneumonia that kills the 33,000 people. The old and the young are at the highest risk, but the secondary complications can happen to anyone in between.

Not everyone can get the flu vaccine, either. You can't get it if you are highly allergic to eggs or any other components of the vaccine. With nine different vaccines currently on the market, you need to ask if you want to know what those components are. For example, gelatin and thimerosal might be two ingredients you'd rather avoid. Not all flu vaccines have them, however, so you have to ask to know for sure.

You *can* get a flu vaccine if you are only somewhat allergic to eggs. Talk to your doctor. Coauthor Chris is among many physicians who now give a percentage (10–50 percent) of the dose initially, then after a waiting period, administer the other percentage (50–90 percent) on the second inoculation. That seems to be tolerated well by those with minor and even some with severe egg allergies. If you have an egg allergy, have your doctor administer the vaccine, not the pharmacist. Some recent medical guidance even states that if you have a non-anaphylactic reaction to eggs, you can get the entire flu vaccine. Either way, talk to your physician.

The other thing that adults and adolescents should get when they come in for their annual flu vaccine is a pertussis booster. Right now the pertussis is combined with the tetanus and that will protect those infants around you from getting the respiratory disease. Adults with whooping cough will have a long, persistent cough and, while it may not kill you, it is a significant irritant to you and everyone around you. Many people complain when they come into a doctor's office with bronchitis, because they have been coughing for two or three weeks. Try *twelve* weeks.

Since 1984, the Advisory Committee on Immunization Practices (ACIP) has recommended that individuals age sixty-five and older should receive pneumococcal polysaccharide vaccine (PPSV). In 2014, ACIP recommended that adults age sixty-five and older should also receive pneumococcal conjugate vaccine (PCV). Therefore, according to ACIP, adults at age sixty-five who have never received pneumococcal vaccine should receive a single dose of PCV13, followed by a dose of PPSV23 six to twelve months later.[12]

A parent's fear of the unknown can be more powerful than the desire to protect. In one instance we rely on denial to make us feel better about our choices; in the other we allow fear to direct our decision making. Science, not fear, is the foundation of the best protection for you and your children. In the discussion of attitudes about vaccination for people of all ages, if we just stay science-centered, we can—someday—have a meeting of the minds.

CHAPTER 5

The Autism Debate

When people get desperate to find an answer to a persistent question—What happens at The Bermuda Triangle? Where is Atlantis? What causes autism?—serious researchers invariably tackle the riddle. And, just as invariably, some of these scientists arrive at conclusions that seem to defy logic. Yet, if their methods are proper, even explanations that sound far-fetched can potentially contribute to ongoing investigations.

Carrie Cariello, author of *What Color is Monday?*, is the mother of an autistic son and a regular contributor to *The Huffington Post*. In the lead-in to her blog post called "I Know What Causes Autism," Cariello laughs at a headline she had just read announcing the link between autism and circumcision.[1]

Since we explored relevant studies for this book, we looked into the source of this headline. It came from ScienceNordic, a website that offers information on the latest research in Nordic countries. Declaring "Study links autism with circumcision," the article notes how a new study "suggests that circumcision increases the risk of developing autism."[2] Published in

the *Journal of the Royal Society of Medicine*, the study did not
reflect some spontaneous act of imaginative scientists, but
rather encompassed a thorough, twenty-year period. The study
involved 342,877 Danish boys born between 1994 and 2003,
who were monitored during the years they were zero to nine
years old.[3] This data was compiled by a senior investigator in epidemiological research and an adjunct professor of sexual health
epidemiology, so at least the team had the "right" credentials.
They speculated that a reason for an autism-circumcision link
is the pain experienced by the newborn during the procedure.
[Note: Circumcision does cause extreme pain when anesthesia
is not used.[4]]

Cariello went on to list a number of other proposed causes or
aggravators of autism that she'd studied over the years. Some she
was clearly spotlighting because she thought they were odd—so
we dug deeper to find out if there was a credible study behind any
of them. The results were surprising:

- **Cause:** Automobile exhaust fumes
  Source: Multiple studies, including those conducted by sepa-
  rate research teams at Columbia and Harvard
- **Cause:** Non-stick cookware
  Source: A study on perfluorinated compounds (PFC) conducted
  by a medical researcher at the Harvard School of Public Health
- **Cause:** Poor maternal bonding
  Source: Several studies, such as one conducted by an interna-
  tional team from multiple universities that presented its
  findings at an Annual Meeting of the Society for Neuroscience
- **Cause:** Plastics
  Source: A study conducted by a team from Rowan University
  and the Rutgers New Jersey School of Medicine on bisphenol A
  (BPA), which is found in some plastics[5]

In light of the multiple reasons given by various researchers about the theorized cause(s) of autism, it is safe to say that the studies and speculation will continue. It is also safe to say that not all conclusions of the studies should be given equal legitimacy and not all will stand the test of time.

Regarding the key studies conducted that explore any link between autism and vaccines, we need to address the disastrous research effort that launched the conversation: Andrew Wakefield's "Ileal-lymphoid-nodular hyperplasia, non-specific colitis and pervasive developmental disorder in children," published February 1998 in *The Lancet*.

On February 2, 2011, National Public Radio's Diane Rehm hosted a discussion of "Vaccines and Autism" that included Alison Singer, president of the Autism Science Foundation, Roberta DeBiasi, a pediatric infectious diseases physician and Seth Mnookin, author of *The Panic Virus: A True Story of Medicine, Science and Fear*. In offering perspective on the scientific method used by Wakefield, the former British physician whose 1998 paper linking vaccines and autism was later discredited, Mnookin said:

> His [Wakefield's] study was based on twelve children, which is called a case series. Even if all of his data had been accurate, drawing a conclusion for a case series would be like saying the four people in this room are a case series and so 75 percent of the population is female.[6]

It's a statement of fact and not a judgment, yet a few callers still suggested that Wakefield's work should not be dismissed. Although many felt his method was flawed, they reasoned, that doesn't mean he was wrong. So despite the fact that many credible studies have indicated that there is no causative relationship between vaccines and autism, doubt still persists.

Two points were made by the panelists that help move us to the debate on vaccines and autism. The first addresses a long-standing philosophical issue in the context of scientific investigation: In the face of recalcitrant data, is a hypothesis still valid? In this case, the unproven theory that studies appear to discount is that something in vaccines or something about vaccination can trigger autism. Alison Singer phrased the conundrum in this manner:

> I think the challenge is that science can never prove a negative. You can never prove definitively that vaccines do not cause autism; you can only show, based on a large body of studies, that vaccines were not related to autism in those studies. Just like similarly, I could climb up to the roof of this building and I could tie a sheet on the back of my head and jump off the building and...if I did it 5,000 times, I would likely land on the ground 5,000 times, but that doesn't prove that I can't fly.[7]

The second point addresses the system of checks and balances inherent to the process of developing a vaccine. In chapter 3, we provided some insights into the development of selected vaccines, noting that in some cases it took decades to come up with a formula that was both safe and effective according to the studies to which it was subjected.

Roberta DeBiasi, the pediatric infectious diseases physician on the panel, gave an overview of how that process works. If there is promising data related to cellular and animal research—and it could take years to accumulate that data—then the company approaches the Food and Drug Administration (FDA), which is tasked with examining the safety and efficacy of food and drugs before they are allowed to come to market. There are more studies and more tests, independent of those conducted by the company developing the product. As a next step:

They have to present some preclinical data in small numbers of people, which are never children, by the way. The studies are always done initially in adults. If there's safety and efficacy, then things finally trickle down to children and this process is anywhere from five, ten, twelve years in the case of varicella vaccine, so I think it is a misunderstanding that some people think pharmaceutical companies can just say "Hey, I've got a vaccine" and we all say "Okay, we're going to use it, it's safe." There's a lot of oversight before we ever recommend giving a vaccine to a child.[8]

To clarify DeBiasi's comment about varicella, that specific vaccine was developed by Merck in 1995, so it had already gone through the initial testing phase just described by that time. However, it was not until 2006 that the vaccine made it onto ACIP's list of recommended immunizations for children.

The problem is: Even if a vaccine goes through years of rigorous testing, with side effects exhaustively examined and thoroughly described, vaccines ultimately end up in people and people are full of surprises. Returning to point number one about recalcitrant data, just because we're almost sure that vaccines don't trigger autism, how can we be positive?

CAUSES OF AUTISM

There are many studies in which researchers directly cite genetics as the cause of autism. But those studies and the mainstream media reports on them do not seem to have much sway on public opinion.

We conducted a survey of our own about this issue, which gives a good sense of what people in America currently think. Among the ten statements we posed requesting a "True" or "False" response was this one: "Genetics are the sole cause of autism." Sixty-five percent of the respondents answered "False" to this statement. Several of the comments indicated that some believed the jury was still out on this issue.

The preponderance of evidence—from both studies and anecdotes—points to a pattern of autism spectrum disorders that runs in families. Researchers are still probing to determine the extent to which metabolic, bio-chemical, neurological and environmental factors also affect the emergence of autism. In our survey, 86 percent of respondents indicated they felt it was true that "Environmental pollutants like auto exhaust are more harmful to children than vaccines." We did not ask them to give an opinion on whether or not these pollutants could cause autism, but there was the clear perception among respondents that environmental hazards threaten our children's health.

The latest science about the causes of autism provides some insights that should have people on both sides of the debate wanting to find out more. The science we want to focus on in this chapter is not the studies about exhaust fumes or attachment issues, although those may well be important factors in the emergence of autism in a child. We want to look at the following two potential causes as precursors to the debate: genetics and vaccines.

The word "autism," which has been in use since the early 1900s, comes from Greek; "autos" means "self," so autism describes conditions in which a person is "an isolated self."[9] The first person to use the term was a Swiss psychiatrist named Eugen Bleuler, who considered it descriptive for a set of schizophrenia symptoms. By the 1940s, the word took on a different meaning, with the medical community in the United States using it in reference to children with various emotional and social problems.

Issues of communication and interaction in autism can range from mild to severe. The symptoms are usually seen early in development, although children with milder types, such as Asperger's syndrome, may not receive a diagnosis until later. One point to be made upfront is that the onset of autism symptoms generally coincides with the time children tend to be getting many of their initial vaccinations. The "causality versus coincidence" argument is, therefore, a key part of the debate.

The explanation of the genetic roots of autism is complicated. It involves inherited variants of genes, as well as mutations of genes that occur in the sperm or egg from which the child was conceived or possibly in the early days of the embryo's development. Instead of going into that, we want to focus on one slice of the research: the MET gene variant.

MET is the common name for a gene called "MET proto-oncogene, receptor tyrosine kinase." If you know a little bit about MET, then you know a few important things about autism and the immune system.

Pat Levitt, PhD, discovered something about MET that should help shape the discussion of autism causes and perhaps the debate over autism and vaccines. Levitt is Simms/Mann Chair in Developmental Neurogenetics Program, Keck School of Medicine, University of Southern California. In addition to his many awards and symposia, he is also an author on 190 peer-reviewed papers throughout his forty-year career. His most recent work covers important ground in the study of autism. Levitt's research is based on a mountain of experience and it does not have a vaccine-related agenda. That's the problem with a lot of people who are quoted—sometimes extensively—online about the link (or lack thereof) between Autism Spectrum Disorders (ASD) and vaccines.

In *Infectious Behavior: Brain-Immune Connections in Autism, Schizophrenia, and Depression*, Paul H. Patterson describes his colleague's key discovery:

> Pat Levitt, now at the Keck School of Medicine at the University of Southern California, found that the presence of a common variant of the gene MET increases the risk for ASD. Levitt also found that the MET protein is reduced in

autism brain samples. The key point for the present discussion is that the MET gene is known to play a role in neuronal development and in the GI tract and is also important in immune system function![10]

Patterson relates this to a type of hypersensitivity found in the immune cells of autistic subjects. He then states:

> Thus, a single gene variant (of MET) or a single environmental insult (maternal infection) can have permanent effects on all three systems—brain, GI and immune.[11]

However, as Levitt clarified for us, we *cannot* interpret this to mean that the gene variant increases the risk that the child will overreact to the antigens in a vaccine. He also expressed concern with drawing any firm conclusion about the impact of the gene variant on immunity in general, because "there have not been any human or animal studies about this."[12]

Careful scientists pull back from stating absolutes, sometimes in the face of abundant studies. That's one reason why their statements often fail to satisfy the general public's desire for a firm answer. Saying that autism has genetic causes is about as firm as it gets in this case. This is fact, although that statement of fact does not leave other factors—metabolic, bio-chemical, neurological and environmental—off the hook.

A challenge in getting a firm answer also relates to who has autism and who may be misdiagnosed as autistic. Genetic investigations called a "microarray" are currently ongoing. Researchers are looking at about 2,000 genes—and the results are all over the place! Many kids diagnosed with "autism" have many non-related gene abnormalities, while others have nothing. Some have sequences that are seen in other autism patients, but nothing specific correlates with the patients' exposure. Some of them are vaccinated on schedule, while others were undervaccinated or not vaccinated at all.

Researchers at the Johns Hopkins Bloomberg School of Public Health looked at more than 1,300 children who had been diagnosed with autism. They found that certain disorders distinguished children who had a current autism diagnosis from those who had "fallen out" of the autism category as they aged. The other "associated disorders" mentioned in the study are learning disability, developmental delay, speech problems, anxiety and seizures or epilepsy. The study suggests that separate diagnoses of learning disabilities or speech problems appeared to predict which kids would continue to be autistic and which ones might grow out of the diagnosis. But were these kids truly autistic in the first place?

The fact that some kids had "fallen out of" or "outgrown" the autism diagnosis shows that perhaps society is overusing the term "autism" to mean a broad spectrum of developmental delays. A person does not "outgrow" a diagnosis of Down's Syndrome or Fragile X and these conditions were present well before the child received any vaccines. Coauthor Chris sees Asperger's patients regularly who are still the same as they always have been; these patients did not "outgrow" their condition. As a physician, Chris asserts that the kids who outgrew their diagnosis had a different underlying cause for their delays entirely.

By overusing the term "autism," it becomes harder to pinpoint what causes true autism. There is a broad set of criteria to look at; with autism overlapping so many other diagnoses, all with many different causes, it's hard to know if we will ever firmly answer the question: "What causes autism?"

THE VACCINE-AUTISM LINK

The theories related to a vaccine-autism link are mainly these, taken from a summary on the topic called "Vaccines and Autism:

A Tale of Shifting Hypotheses" by two leading physicians in the Division of Infectious Diseases at The Children's Hospital of Philadelphia:

1. The combination measles-mumps-rubella vaccine causes autism by damaging the intestinal lining, which allows the entrance of encephalopathic proteins.

2. Thimerosal, an ethylmercury-containing preservative in some vaccines, is toxic to the central nervous system.

3. The simultaneous administration of multiple vaccines overwhelms or weakens the immune system.[13]

In the remainder of this chapter (and in the subsequent chapter on vaccine additives), we will explore these three theories and the contrasting assertions related to them.

WHERE ARE WE WITH THE STUDIES?

In a 2011 article for *The Huffington Post*, model and autism activist Jenny McCarthy packed one paragraph more than others with multiple concerns and assertions. It's a good paragraph to introduce a state-of-the-studies discussion—in which we review the research and analysis that has been performed by both sides or is currently going on.

> I know children regress after vaccination because it happened to my own son. Why aren't there any tests out there on the safety of how vaccines are administered in the real world, six at a time? Why have only two of the thirty-six shots our kids receive been looked at for their relationship to autism? Why hasn't anyone ever studied completely non-vaccinated children to understand their autism rate?[14]

The key points McCarthy makes are about regression, the simultaneous administration of vaccines, a comprehensive look at vaccine-autism relationships and autism rates in vaccinated versus unvaccinated children. Here is current information on studies in each of those four areas.

REGRESSION

Autism Speaks has funded a "vaccination with regression study," which is currently ongoing as of this writing. The challenge that researchers have faced comes from observing regression immediately or shortly after vaccination. There are simply no procedures or tests in place to identify the phenomenon that parents like Jenny McCarthy describe, so the information has been primarily anecdotal.

The study involves the Atlanta, Georgia, Kaiser Permanente electronic database, which helps researchers identify children with regressive types of autism. They are trying to connect their condition to the timing of vaccination, with a particular focus on the MMR vaccine. What they are looking for is a concentration of visits post-vaccination—tests, procedures, parental reports of health changes, etc. They are reviewing emergency room visits in the day or two after vaccination, along with any notes on crying, irritability, fever and other symptoms of problems. The database will also have information on test results from CT scans on the children, any metabolic testing that was done and the nature of referrals to specialists such as neurologists.

However, their analysis should be viewed as the beginning of a process. Whatever they come up with will help other researchers in their designs of studies with specific populations.

Frustrated parents have been crying out for years that their stories about regression after vaccination have been discredited by the medical establishment. A prime assertion of the medical community is that the timing of vaccinations coincides with the time

when autism symptoms tend to surface, so it's a matter of coincidence, not causality. The Kaiser Permanente study won't give definitive answers, but it could help move the conversation forward.

SIMULTANEOUS ADMINISTRATION OF VACCINES

A number of studies have been conducted to investigate the
effects of giving simultaneous combinations of vaccines. More
importantly, those studies are part of an ongoing process. All vaccines are subjected to concomitant studies when the companies
seek approval to bring them to market, meaning that the new
vaccines are tested in conjunction with existing ones to make sure
the combination is safe.

The overarching concern that some parents have is that there
are so many vaccines administered to infants that their immune
systems get overwhelmed and/or there are negative neurological
repercussions. That assertion is addressed in the following sections,
with the case of Hannah Poling receiving particular attention.
It's a landmark case, because it centers on how a child with a
pre-existing condition is traumatized by the same number of vaccinations that another child would have little or no response to.

With the great majority of children, the reality is quite different from Hannah Poling's case. Bacteria encountered all day
long constantly keep the immune system on alert. It's not usually
something that a person would notice, but it's there all the same.
Just feel the lymph nodes on a toddler's neck; they are always
lumpy. He or she is always fighting something and the body performs more effectively when it is prepared ahead of time. It is a
body that knows what to do with the small amounts of antigens
in the vaccines.

COMPREHENSIVE LOOK AT VACCINE-AUTISM RELATIONSHIPS

McCarthy asks, "Why have only two of the thirty-six shots children receive been looked at for their relationship to autism?" This

assumption is flawed. First of all, any vaccine that now contains thimerosal or used to contain thimerosal fell under the scrutiny of researchers looking for an autism-vaccine link. Currently, three different types of vaccines given to children contain thimerosal: some brands of influenza vaccine, one type of tetanus/diphtheria vaccine (not the combination vaccines containing DTaP) and one type of meningococcal vaccine. In previous years, there were others, including MMR.

Secondly, in September 2014 a pro-life website called LifeNews.com announced that a new study linked autism to any vaccines made with cells from aborted fetuses. They targeted MMR, varicella (chickenpox) and hepatitis A vaccines. The study called "Impact of environmental factors on the prevalence of autistic disorder after 1979" was funded by Sound Choice Pharmaceutical Institute and published in the *Journal of Public Health and Epidemiology* that month. (In all fairness to McCarthy, this study came out after her comment was published in *The Huffington Post*.)

Joseph Mercola, a well-known alternative medicine proponent and vaccination opponent, says various analyses of trends in the United States, Denmark and Israel will link Hib vaccine to the dramatic rise in autism cases.[15]

AUTISM RATES IN VACCINATED VERSUS UNVACCINATED CHILDREN

In her final question, McCarthy asks: "Why hasn't anyone ever studied completely non-vaccinated children to understand their autism rate?" A response to this question is "How?" Researchers have already tried to the extent that is possible, but there are huge challenges in studying children as opposed to just analyzing data about them.

In their 2009 paper, "Vaccines and Autism: A Tale of Shifting Hypotheses," Jeffrey Gerber and Paul Offit describe the challenge in these words:

> No studies have compared the incidence of autism in vacci-
> nated, unvaccinated or alternatively vaccinated children (i.e.,
> schedules that spread out vaccines, avoid combination vac-
> cines or include only select vaccines). These studies would be
> difficult to perform because of the likely differences among
> these three groups in healthcare seeking behavior and the eth-
> ics of experimentally studying children who have not received
> vaccines.[16]

The authors don't suggest it's impossible to do what McCarthy proposes. But it would seem to require cooperation between parents who have pulled back from the ACIP vaccination schedule and researchers from the medical establishment. Or vice versa. How likely is that?

The people who question vaccine safety and/or reject vaccination offer data analyses that assert unvaccinated children have lower rates of autism. Unsurprisingly, data analyses cited by those in the pro-vaccination camp conclude that autism rates between vaccinated and unvaccinated children do not vary in a statistically significant way.

The International Medical Council on Vaccination compared autism rates in a vaccinated population to rates in an Amish community; their premise is that the Amish children are an unvaccinated population. According to their website, the Council "is an association of medical doctors, registered nurses and other qualified medical professionals whose purpose is to counter the messages asserted by pharmaceutical companies, the government and medical agencies that vaccines are safe, effective and harmless."[17]

The contrast they expressed is that, in the general population of children in the United States, one in 100 is diagnosed with autism. This is the number associated with the "vaccinated" population. The "unvaccinated" population they cited was the Amish community of Lancaster County, Pennsylvania. With regards to this population, the Council noted the following: one in 4,875 diagnosed with autism.[18]

These numbers come from the Age of Autism website (one in 100) and an ad hoc survey of Lancaster County Amish (one in 4,875) conducted by Dan Olmstead, editor of the Age of Autism website. The figure commonly used today by the Autism Society and CDC is actually more shocking than the Council's one in 100: It's one in sixty-eight.

The reference to the Amish community is also incorrect. The underlying premise is that the Amish of Lancaster County do not vaccinate their children but, in fact, they do. In an article posted on the "Discover Lancaster" website, there are plenty of insights into the Pennsylvania Amish community, including their style of transportation, language, recreation, dress and health, among other things. The Amish are plagued with certain genetic diseases (though they have avoided many others), so they have been the subject of focused studies by nearby universities, including the University of Maryland. That is to say, medical researchers are keeping an eye on them and know how they manage certain health-related issues.

Regarding the Lancaster County Amish vaccination rate, the frontline source of information is the Clinic for Special Children in Strasburg, Pennsylvania, which specializes in serving the health needs of the Amish in the area. Dr. Kevin Strauss at the Clinic says, "The Amish do vaccinate their children. Their overall vaccination rate is lower in comparison to the general populace, but you'll find a higher rate of vaccination among young Amish than in older generations. The bi-weekly vaccination clinic that we run is very busy."[19]

The perception that the Amish don't vaccinate their children was something we heard over and over again, so we included the following statement in our survey and asked for a "True" or "False" response: "The Amish do not vaccinate their children." Sixty-four percent of the respondents agreed with the statement. One of the respondents who answered "False" gave a thoughtful comment: "In such a tight-knit community, an introduction of a disease like measles would be disastrous, so I would think that they vaccinate."

Discrepancies aside, the kind of numbers cited could well point to some real differences, but the only way to confirm or deny the conclusion is to do what McCarthy suggested and study vaccinated versus unvaccinated populations. This is what a Japanese team from the Yokahama Rehabilitation Center did.

In Japan, the MMR vaccine was introduced in 1989, but the country stopped using it in 1993 as the Japanese moved to a single-vaccine program. This gave Japanese scientists the unique opportunity to study autism rates in two distinct populations: those who received the MMR vaccine and those who did not. If there were a link between MMR and autism, the number of autism diagnoses should have plummeted after the withdrawal of the MMR vaccine. They didn't; they went up just as they did in the United States and in other countries around the world.

The study examined the incidences of ASD in an area of Japan with a population of about 300,000 people. The researchers considered every child diagnosed with ASD born between 1986 and 1996, up to age seven. After seeing a rise in autism rates after MMR was withdrawn, their conclusion was simply that MMR is not the likely cause of ASD.[20]

We want to emphasize that MMR was the only vaccine considered in this study. If one or more other vaccines might play a role in the onset of autism, that possibility was not covered by this Japanese research.

In a slightly different take on the issue, with many of the study participants being undervaccinated rather than unvaccinated, the University of California-Davis MIND Institute compared the immunization practices of preschoolers with ASD and what is called "typical development." The Institute's work holds an interesting place in this discussion, since it was founded in 1998 by families dealing with autism and has gained the respect of groups that generally espouse the notion that there is a link between autism and vaccines.

The team from the MIND Institute presented their findings at the International Meeting for Autism Research in May 2013. The title declares: "No Differences in Early Immunization Rates among Children with Typical Development and Autism Spectrum Disorders." This was a relatively small study involving 240 children, but a high number of participants—161 of them—were children diagnosed with ASD and part of the MIND Institute's Autism Phenome Project. Immunization rates in ASD children were slightly *lower* than in the typical development group, but the team did not consider the difference statistically significant. One of the ASD children had never received any vaccinations. The team asserted that their work "did not support an association between vaccines and ASD."[21]

When the Institute's findings were summarized on the AutismWeb Forum site, many readers criticized the study as an oversimplification. Their frustration was palpable: Once again, research they felt was flawed asserted they were "wrong" in seeing a connection between vaccines and the autism in their children. They called for even more studies, especially cross-disciplinary ones involving genetics, toxicology and systems biology.[22]

ASSERTION: VACCINES CAUSE AUTISM

The community that rejects vaccines completely (or at least in part) cites long lists of studies they believe help prove the autism-vaccine link. These are the key topic areas that we have seen addressed in those studies:

- Hepatitis B vaccine and autism in boys
- Aluminum and autism

- Thimerosal and autism
- Vaccination triggering regression in children with certain metabolic problems
- Vaccines and brain inflammation
- Vaccine toxicity and autism

As expected, each topic was criticized by scientists who found fault with the study designs, data analysis or some other aspect of the work they felt discredited the findings. The arguments for and against are many and complex. What the community of vaccine critics has long been looking for is someone from inside the medical/pharmaceutical/research establishment—someone held in high regard by that community—to step out and say, "We got it wrong. Vaccines are a problem."

On August 27, 2014, these vaccine critics got their wish. CDC Senior Scientist William Thompson issued a press release confirming rumors of his allegations that the CDC had withheld information about an autism-vaccine link. He did not go public with his statement until a colleague unmasked him after secretly taping conversations about the study results. Thompson said,

> I regret that my coauthors and I omitted statistically significant information in our 2004 article published in the journal *Pediatrics*. The omitted data suggested that African-American males who received the MMR vaccine before age thirty-six months were at increased risk for autism. Decisions were made regarding which findings to report after the data were collected and I believe that the final study protocol was not followed.
>
> ...My concern has been the decision to omit relevant findings in a particular study for a particular sub-group for a particular vaccine. There have always been recognized risks for vaccination and I believe it is the responsibility of the CDC

to properly convey the risks associated with receipt of those vaccines.[23]

More than ten years before that statement, Thompson had sent a letter to Julie Gerberding, the CDC director at the time. In the letter, Thompson expressed concern about what he was going to say at an upcoming Institute of Medicine Meeting: "I will be presenting the summary of our results from the Metropolitan Atlanta Autism Case-Control Study and I will have to present several problematic results relating to statistical associations between the receipt of MMR vaccine and autism."[24] In receiving official whistleblower status, Thompson retains his position with the CDC and is free to testify before Congress about the matter; a hearing date has not been scheduled as of this writing.

In addition to the Thompson assertion, ostensibly one of the strongest arguments that there is a tie between vaccines and neurological conditions falling within the autism spectrum is that damages have been awarded to parents for vaccine injury. The non-profit organization National Vaccine Information Center (NVIC) funds research on vaccine safety and provides assistance to people who maintain that they or members of their family have suffered from vaccine reactions. The group's founders worked with Congress to craft and pass the National Childhood Vaccine Injury Act of 1986, which led to a procedure for filing claims and financially compensating injured parties. In 1988, the law enabled the creation of the National Vaccine Injury Compensation Program (VICP). The US Court of Federal Claims decides who will be paid, but the US Department of Health and Human Services and the Department of Justice are also involved in the process.

One case that put the spotlight on a link between autism and vaccination involved an Atlanta girl named Hannah Poling. Her father happens to be a neurologist. Her mother is a registered nurse.

Hannah did not appear to have symptoms of autism during her first eighteen months of life. At that point, she received the vaccines for measles, mumps, rubella, polio, varicella, diphtheria, pertussis, tetanus and Hib. Afterwards, she had high fevers and a lack of appetite, eventually withdrawing into an uncommunicative state. She also had screaming fits. Two years later, Hannah's parents filed a claim. In 2010, the government settled the case before trial and the Polings were awarded $1.5 million as compensation for Hannah's injuries. In CBS's coverage of the Poling case, investigative journalist Sharyl Attkisson had this to say:

> In acknowledging Hannah's injuries, the government said vaccines aggravated an unknown mitochondrial disorder Hannah had which didn't "cause" her autism, but "resulted" in it. It's unknown how many other children have similar undiagnosed mitochondrial disorder. All other autism "test cases" have been defeated at trial. Approximately 4,800 are awaiting disposition in federal vaccine court.[25]

The mitochondrial disorder to which the statement refers means that Hannah has a dysfunction in basic cell metabolism. The variations on this kind of disorder mean that the symptoms can vary greatly.

Interestingly, Julie Gerberding, the director at CDC when William Thompson expressed concerns over his autism-vaccine findings in 2004, also held that title throughout the Poling case. Her comment to reporters about the decision was this: "The government has made absolutely no statement indicating that vaccines are a cause for autism."[26]

Parents who want an answer regarding any impact that vaccines might have on causing or triggering autism think that kind of dismissal is lame.

ASSERTION: VACCINES DO NOT CAUSE AUTISM

Aggravation of a pre-existing condition is not the same as causing the condition. Medical research by a diverse group of scientists points to genetics as the actual cause of autism. Among the many researchers who examined the genetic basis of autism are teams from the following US institutes and university departments, as well as researchers from Poland, Japan and many other nations:

- J. Drexel Autism Institute, Drexel University
- Keck School of Medicine, University of Southern California
- Center for Autism Research and Treatment, Semel Institute, David Geffen School of Medicine, University of California
- Johns Hopkins University School of Medicine
- Biological & Biomedical Sciences, Yale University
- National Institute of Neuroscience, National Institutes of Health
- Oregon Health & Science University
- UCLA Mindful Awareness Research Center

Their work does not preclude the possibility that factors other than genetics are in play, however. As stated before, plenty of studies have also looked at environmental factors and included research done to ascertain any impact of vaccines on children. But there is a big difference between saying "vaccines cause autism" and "a child with risk factors for ASD may respond differently to vaccines."

A statement like that doesn't take the heat off of pharmaceutical companies or government organizations when it comes to vaccine safety—or at least it shouldn't. It points to a new level of responsibility. If it really is likely that a child with a certain gene variant could have a horrible reaction to a vaccine, then the challenge is identifying the problem before the vaccine is administered, not blaming the vaccine for the problem.

In light of the premise that the cause of autism appears to be genetic, let's revisit the three primary types of assertions related to a possible vaccine-autism link:

- MMR vaccine causes autism by damaging the intestinal lining, which was Wakefield's assertion.
- Thimerosal is toxic to the central nervous system.
- Giving several vaccines at once overwhelms or weakens the immune system.

Turning first to the assertion that the MMR vaccine causes autism, there is an abundance of studies on the issue. Roberta DeBiasi, referred to earlier for her participation in the NPR panel on vaccines and autism, rebutted one of the callers to the show who felt that Wakefield's premise—not the study itself—had been undervalued:

> In the case of the Wakefield theory, there has been a debate. And that's come in the form of twenty-four studies from five countries that have all shown the same thing…So I'm a little baffled why people think his theory has been ignored. It's been actually looked at very closely.

The "same thing" to which DeBiasi refers is the refutation that there is any link between the MMR vaccine and autism, particularly as it pertains to GI tract involvement. But who performed these studies and why does the pro-vax community put so much stock in them? Here is a sampling of the studies that were launched relatively soon after Wakefield's paper was published.

The terms describing these studies are used to inform other scientists of the study population and methods. What this indicates is that there are different types of studies that reached the same conclusion and that they were all considered far more vigorous and reliable models than Wakefield's.

STUDIES THAT FAIL TO SUPPORT AN ASSOCIATION BETWEEN MEASLES-MUMPS-RUBELLA AND AUTISM

SOURCE	STUDY DESIGN	STUDY LOCATION
Taylor et al., 1999	Ecological	United Kingdom
Farrington et al., 2001	Ecological	United Kingdom
Kaye et al., 2001	Ecological	United Kingdom
Dales et al., 2006	Ecological	United States
Fombonne et al., 2006	Ecological	Canada
Fombonne and Chakrabarti, 2001	Ecological	United Kingdom
Taylor et al., 2002	Ecological	United Kingdom
DeWilde et al., 2001	Case-control	United Kingdom
Makela et al., 2002	Retrospective cohort	Finland
Madsen et al., 2002	Retrospective cohort	Denmark
DeStafano et al., 2004	Case-control	United States
Peltola et al., 1998	Prospective cohort	Finland
Patja et al., 2000	Prospective cohort	Finland

Stanley Plotkin et al. *Clinical Infectious Diseases* 2009; 48:456-461

Earlier in the chapter, we noted that Wakefield's study was called a case series. A case series is descriptive in nature and, as the name suggests, it looks at a series of cases. Conversely, a cohort study is far more robust: "A cohort study, in principle, enables the calculation of an absolute risk or a rate for the outcome; such a calculation is not possible in a case series."[27] A cohort study is one type of observational study, which is often used when it may not be ethical to do a controlled trial. Rather than ask the parents of 50,000 kids not to give their children the MMR vaccine so they could be placed in a control group and studied alongside 50,000 kids who got the vaccine—most physicians would have ethics issues with that—the researchers go on observation.

For example, the paper "Autism occurrence by MMR vaccine status among US children with older siblings with and without autism" was published in *JAMA* in April 2015. It's a cohort study involving 95,727 children that concluded: "These findings indicate no harmful association between MMR vaccine receipt and ASD even among children already at higher risk for ASD."[28] Recall that Wakefield's case series involved just twelve children.

Like a cohort study, case-control and ecological studies are observational. The subjects in a case-control study are defined as cases and controls; researchers compare exposure histories to something like thimerosal, for example. Ecological studies involve a large database, so the investigation of a relationship between exposure and outcome is at a population level. There are also other types of studies, but the key point is that critics of a conclusion often focus on the study design for its shortcomings or strengths. Those in the research community should acknowledge that there are both advantages and disadvantages to each type of design. Prospective cohort studies tend to be very expensive, for example, because they follow subjects over time.

One of the things we've seen over and over again is apples-and-oranges comparisons of studies about autism and vaccines. So if you do want to have a debate involving dueling studies, do the homework first to find out who was studied, over what period of time, whether or not there were control subjects and how the data analysis was conducted.

Citing Wakefield's work as an important study is a difficult proposition, not just because of the type of study, but also because of some inherent flaws. His central premise is that the MMR vaccine caused intestinal inflammation which led to "translocation of unusually nonpermeable peptides to the bloodstream and, subsequently, to the brain, where they affected development."[29] For that to be plausible, one would deduce that all of the eight ASD kids in his study group of twelve would have gastrointestinal symptoms first and then experience the onset of autism. That was not the case in the group.

The issue of thimerosal and toxicity is explored in greater depth in the next chapter. Here, we will simply say that the AAP asked for the immediate removal of thimerosal from any vaccines given to infants in 1999—right after the FDA determined how much mercury children might be receiving in their first six months of life from various sources. That decision was precautionary and extremely conservative, since they didn't have evidence that thimerosal was actually a problem. Nonetheless, many parents saw that action as a red flag.

Having already presented the unfortunate case of Hannah Poling in relation to a rare effect of giving multiple vaccinations at once, we'll now look at why most of the medical community doesn't see this as a problem. The argument is that giving several vaccines at once overwhelms or weakens the immune system. The reality is:

- Even tiny human bodies—and this does presume the infants are basically healthy—can generate the protective responses required to handle multiple vaccines. There are also studies suggesting they could take a great deal more than they are currently receiving on the schedule.
- One reason why they could receive a lot more is that vaccines aren't the same as they used to be in the twentieth century. The fourteen vaccines given early in a child's life today contain fewer than 200 immunological components, whereas the seven vaccines that kids got in 1980 contained more than 3,000 of these components.

Thus, three of the prime arguments that suggest something other than genetics causes autism have significant weaknesses. They also point to legitimate reasons why we need to examine the possibility that something in vaccines or the vaccination process itself might cause a child with a pre-existing condition to react badly.

We want to add one more bit of science to this debate, which relates to how a mother might take steps to avert autism. This has nothing to do with avoiding vaccines, but rather taking care of herself. Using data from the "Norwegian Mother and Child Cohort Study" published on March 12, 2014, a *Journal of the American Medical Association* (JAMA) study found that mothers who took folic acid four weeks before and during the first eight weeks of pregnancy had a 40 percent reduced risk of having a child with autism.[30] The study followed over 85,000 babies born between 2002–2008 and their parents' vitamin intake, among other things. The mothers reported whether they were taking folic acid before and during early pregnancy prior to finding out whether their children had a diagnosis of autism.

About 270 babies of parents in this study were born with a developmental disorder on the autism spectrum. That's a rate of 0.003 percent risk, which is far lower than our 2015 listed rates of one in sixty-eight (0.015 percent). Physicians already counsel mothers to take folic acid in order to prevent spina bifida, a neural tube defect. So we see a low rate of autism in parents who took simple measures to reduce one neurological issue; the same simple measures can reduce the risk of what is likely another neurological issue, autism.

The lists of studies on both sides of the autism-vaccine debate are so long that any parent would find it almost impossible to sort out the science. What we have tried to do here is ask those who care about the debate to acknowledge that there are plenty of "maybes" and "what ifs." Scientific research thrives on both, so the hope is that we will have even longer lists of studies in the near future and that some will lead to important conclusions.

CHAPTER 6

The Additives and Preservatives Debate

Vaccines contain more than the virus or bacterium that serves as the main ingredient. Some of these other substances are at the heart of the controversy over vaccine safety.

The various types of substances commonly used in the production of vaccines include:

- A suspending fluid, which might be sterile water, saline or fluid containing protein.
- Preservatives and stabilizers. Some of these include the substances on which anti-vaxxers focus, like thimerosal. A few of the many others are:
    o Albumin, a simple protein such as egg white, that is water-soluble. The concern centers on an allergy to eggs.
    o Phenol, a common disinfectant. If you read the Merriam-Webster Dictionary definition you might be alarmed as well: "a corrosive poisonous crystalline acidic compound C_6H_5OH present in the tars of coal and wood that in dilute solution is used as a disinfectant."[1]

o   Glycine, a nonessential amino acid. According to WebMD,
     glycine is "safe for most people."[2] Though not a rousing
     endorsement, it does make the substance appear benign.
- Enhancers that help improve the vaccine's effectiveness.
- In some vaccines, there are very small amounts of the culture
  material used to grow the virus or bacteria, such as chicken egg
  protein.

A vaccine described earlier in terms of the "when" and "why"
of it is DTaP-Hep B-IPV. This vaccine protects against five different
childhood diseases: diphtheria, hepatitis B, pertussis (whooping
cough), polio and tetanus. As mentioned before, it's given in
a series of injections, the first of which is usually administered
when the child is two months old. Booster shots are then given
at four and six months of age. GlaxoSmithKline makes this particular vaccine, known commercially as Pediarix, although there
are other similar combination vaccines.

You might assume that this vaccine contains quite a few substances since it protects a child from five different diseases—and
it does contain more ingredients than many other vaccines on
the market today. The inactive ingredients, known as excipients,
of Pediarix are listed as:

- Formaldehyde
- Glutaraldehyde
- Aluminum hydroxide
- Aluminum phosphate
- Lactalbumin hydrolysate
- Polysorbate 80
- Neomycin sulfate
- Polymyxin B
- Yeast protein
- Calf serum

- Fenton medium (containing bovine extract)
- Modified Latham medium (derived from bovine casein)
- Modified Stainer-Scholte liquid medium
- Vero (monkey kidney) cells[3]

It's important to note that this is not only the list of inactive ingredients found in Pediarix, but also the substances used during the vaccine's manufacturing process. In some cases, these substances are removed from the final product, but because they may remain in trace quantities, they are still listed here. Sodium Chloride (table salt) is also present in most vaccines.

So let's start with the point of view of a new mother who has been exposed to compelling anecdotal information about the dangers of vaccines. She hasn't read the studies and she hasn't taken chemistry courses since junior year of high school. She asks the pediatrician for a list of ingredients in the vaccine about to be given to her two-month-old baby. The list of excipients we just provided is what she reads.

"Formaldehyde? You're injecting my baby with formaldehyde?" she questions anxiously. The presence of a substance many women associate with nail polish and embalming dead bodies is used in twenty-three different vaccines.[4] To make matters worse, perhaps this new mom was reading an article called "Government Says 2 Common Materials Pose Risk of Cancer" in *The New York Times* one day while she was pregnant; she remembers that the government listed formaldehyde as a known carcinogen.[5] Combine her limited knowledge of chemistry with a recent memory of a negative news report and anecdotes about the dangers of vaccines and you can easily see why we need a discussion about additives and preservatives.

Let's just take a quick look at formaldehyde, because this substance can readily be explained as "safe." Inhaled formaldehyde comes from nasty sources like car exhaust, tobacco smoke and wood stoves. We also ingest it, albeit in very small amounts, from eating apples, carrots, pears, milk and many other foods. Now for the surprise: Our bodies make formaldehyde; it's an essential part of our normal metabolism, required for the synthesis of DNA and amino acids, which are the building blocks of protein.

In vaccines, formaldehyde is used to inactivate viruses so that they don't cause disease. It also serves to detoxify bacterial toxins, such as the one used to make diphtheria vaccine. The Children's Hospital of Philadelphia's Vaccine Education Center offers the following note to parents about formaldehyde in vaccines:

> Assuming an average weight of a two-month-old of 5 kg and an average blood volume of 85 ml per kg, the total quantity of formaldehyde found in an infant's circulation would be about 1.1 mg, a value at least five-fold greater than that to which an infant would be exposed in vaccines.[6]

This substance performs an important function in making the vaccine itself safe. The human body knows what to do with it when taken into the system in tiny amounts as part of a vaccination.

Another substance is the "corrosive poisonous crystalline acidic compound" phenol. An Internet search on the function of phenol in vaccines yields the following bit of *mis*information—which is only available on non-scientific websites that criticize the efficacy of vaccines: "Phenol is included in vaccines to help stimulate immune response."[7] That's not what it does. Phenol is a preservative, now preferred in some cases to thimerosal. Not to be glib, but if you read a standard description of hydrogen, you'd see this: "a colorless, highly flammable element."[8] You drink H_2O every day without bursting into flames, so a basic knowledge of chemistry is, once again, helpful in preventing overreaction to the basic description of a substance.

Preservatives and stabilizers enable vaccines to remain unchanged when they're exposed to heat, light, acidity or humidity. Preservatives are not, by their nature, "good" or "good for you" and research continues to try to determine the most benign preservatives for medical applications. In the meantime, if there is enough evidence of safety issues and/or very loud protests from consumers, substances like thimerosal will continue to be studied and swapped out for the next best thing—in this case, phenol.

WHEN IS A PRESERVATIVE NOT A PRESERVATIVE?

People are concerned about preservatives in vaccines, but *adjuvants* are what some actually refer to when they talk about this topic. The intended role of adjuvants is to provide more antibodies and prolong the vaccine's protection by boosting the immune system's response to the virus or bacteria agent. This occurs without your body developing immunity to the adjuvant itself.

The inactivated type of vaccine requires adjuvants to stimulate an immune response. This is partly why it's possible to reduce the number of actual antigens from the viruses and bacteria needed to make the vaccine, but still get effective protection. In the 1960s, there were about 3,000 antigens in a pertussis (whooping cough) vaccination. Now there are five. As we noted in the previous chapter on the autism debate, by 1980 the seven vaccines given in the first months of life contained more than 3,000 immunological components, whereas the total for today's fourteen vaccines has dropped below 200. The addition of adjuvants is the reason why.

Different studies have observed that adjuvants exert their immune enhancement function in some very basic ways.[9] First, the adjuvants help bring the antigen to the lymph node for processing.

Then they protect the antigen for a little longer, which gives the body more time to form immune factors and enact a stronger response. The adjuvants also cause a greater local reaction at the site; this inflammation brings more immune cells into the area to see what's going on and ultimately "remember" for later exposure.

The choice of adjuvant or immune enhancer determines whether the immune response is effective, ineffective or damaging. Aluminum compounds are typically used in humans and are generally regarded as safe.

ALUMINUM: SHOULD YOU INJECT IT IN YOUR KID?

Robert W. Sears, MD, has become well known for advocating a vaccination schedule that deviates from that of the American Academy of Pediatrics. Part of his reasoning behind the proposal of an alternate schedule is the aluminum content in vaccines. In fact, Sears devotes thirteen pages of his book to this discussion, centering his cautions on the total micrograms of aluminum a baby would receive if the vaccination schedule were followed as prescribed. In the final chapter of *The Vaccine Book*, he details a vaccine schedule that "allows you to get every vaccine in a timely manner, while getting only one aluminum-containing vaccine at a time."[10] If you had no knowledge of why the current vaccination schedule is constructed the way it is (which we explained earlier in this book), then Sears' recommendation sounds rather rational.

The salient point here is linked to a statement that Sears makes very early in his book: "...Some studies indicate that when too many aluminum-containing vaccines are given at once, toxic effects can occur."[11] The problem is there don't appear to be any such studies. An online search for scholarly work on the issue of aluminum in vaccines and potential toxic effects yields results that point to this conclusion: The amount of aluminum used in vaccines is well within safety limits and the prescribed schedule doesn't involve exceeding those limits. As a corollary, aluminum works well as an adjuvant.

However, there is a study published four years after Sears' book that accuses aluminum in vaccines of causing autism and autoimmune disease. The study is called "Aluminum Vaccine Adjuvants: Are they Safe?"[12] and it appears in the *Current Medicinal Chemistry* journal. The authors are Lucija Tomljenovic and Christopher Shaw, two academics who are well-known in the anti-vaccination community.

Several scientists on the other side of the vaccination debate wrote articles attempting to debunk the work of Tomljenovic and Shaw in this study. The most compelling and thorough comes from the CDC's Immunization Safety Assessment working group, which stated:

> On review, the CDC-CISA working group identified scientific concerns with the article, primarily, interpretation of histopathology and immunopathology methods. These concerns negate the authors' conclusions and significantly limit any interpretation of the results shown in the paper.[13]

After this, the working group's technical report cited four "key limitations" in the publication. These limitations aren't just mildly critical; they are damning.

Most people in the United States probably come into contact with aluminum every day. Touching aluminum pans and foil and drinking soda out of aluminum cans are common occurrences for Americans. We crush the can and toss it into the recycling bin, never giving the slightest thought to the supposed toxicity of aluminum. Absorption of aluminum from the soda that's been in the can or the aluminum found in some antiperspirants has caused some people to change their habits, though. There are plenty of alternatives available, so despite the lack of scientific evidence that aluminum poses a problem in these substances, people can play "better safe than sorry" and choose something else.

When it comes to the use of aluminum for medicinal purposes, some form of aluminum is used as part of antiulceratives, astringents, antiseptics, antiperspirants, antimicrobials, analgesics, antacids, antidiarrheal compounds, antifungal medications, dental cement, diaper rash treatments, in food packaging, as a drug coloring agent and in some topical drugs like acne medication. This is in addition to its use as a vaccine adjuvant.

In terms of the micrograms used in vaccines—a microgram is 1/1000 of a milligram—perhaps the most dramatic negative effect is described in this excerpt from a paper in the *Journal of Toxicology and Environmental Health*: "Sensitization has occurred after injection of aluminum-adjuvant-containing vaccines and pollen extracts, resulting in persistent granuloma at the injection site."[14] In other words, you might see inflammation on the skin; it's an immune system response.

If a two-month-old baby receives a shot of Pediarix, the vaccine described earlier in this chapter, there are 850 micrograms (or .85 milligrams) of aluminum substances in one shot designed to protect against five diseases. Let's say the two-month-old baby weighs eleven pounds—that's about five kilograms or five *billion* micrograms. More meaningfully, in terms of studies conducted on the safety limits of aluminum in vaccines, the amount of vaccine adjuvant in Pediarix is one-fifth of the FDA recommended allowance (4.225 milligrams) in that first year of your child's life.[15] Combined with the hepatitis B vaccination given at birth and another month later, the total amount of aluminum a child would likely receive as a vaccine adjuvant in the first years of life is 3.05 milligrams, which is well under the allowable limit.

There is something else to point out here: The article on the FDA website that discusses the recommended maximum allowance of aluminum is titled "Study Reports Aluminum in Vaccines Poses Extremely Low Risk to Infants." That is not the same as "no risk." Despite the research "confirming that the benefits of aluminum-containing vaccines administered during the first year of life outweigh any theoretical concerns about the potential effect of aluminum on infants,"[16] anxious parents might still worry about the lack of an absolute statement of safety. However, researchers with a sound scientific method and intellectual curiosity are not foolish enough to toss around absolutes when it comes to the human body.

THIMEROSAL: WORTH THE FIGHT?

A search for thimerosal-related studies in the PubMed database of the US National Library of Medicine, National Institutes of Health, yields 101 results in such major publications as the *Journal of Pediatric Pharmacology and Therapeutics*, *Pediatrics* and the *American Journal of Preventative Medicine*. Those results also include studies debunked by the overwhelming majority of researchers, such as the work done by Mark and David Geier, which was published in *Medical Science Monitor*. It's important to note that *Medical Science Monitor* was among several publications banned by Thomson Reuters in 2012 for colluding with two other journals to boost their impact ratings by citing each other's articles.[17]

Some high profile individuals, albeit not scientists, have tried to sound the alarm about thimerosal. In some cases, as with Jenny McCarthy, the shots fired are anecdotal horror stories. That is why anti-vaxxers were happy to have Robert F. Kennedy, Jr. on board as a strong critic of thimerosal, based on scientific evidence.

Many people listen when Kennedy speaks on a topic. No one disputes the fact that he's well-known, but he wants to be perceived as someone who does his research and leads the charge on debunking junk science. One set of scientific arguments, to which Kennedy devoted an entire book, asserts that there is a link between autism and exposure to the preservative thimerosal.

To better set up this discussion, it helps to have a definition of the substance in question:

> Thimerosal is a mercury-containing organic compound (an organomercurial). Since the 1930s, it has been widely used as a preservative in a number of biological and drug products, including many vaccines, to help prevent potentially life threatening contamination with harmful microbes.[18]

On July 7, 1999, the American Academy of Pediatrics and the US Public Health Service issued a joint statement recommending the removal of thimerosal from manufactured vaccines. Their action was partly prompted by an FDA risk assessment, which consisted of hazard identification, dose-response assessment, exposure assessment and risk characterization. The big question was: Is thimerosal toxic and, if so, at what dose does toxicity occur? There are two important facts related to this question. The first is that ethylmercury is a metabolite of thimerosal, meaning it's a product of metabolic action after thimerosal is introduced into the body. Second, methylmercury is a similar organic mercury compound.

The CDC makes the distinction in these terms:

- **Methylmercury** is formed in the environment when mercury metal is present. If this material is found in the body, it is usually the result of eating some types of fish or other food. High amounts of methylmercury can harm the nervous system. This has been found in studies of some populations that have long-term exposure to methylmercury in foods at levels that are far higher than the US population. In the United States, federal guidelines keep as much methylmercury as possible out of the environment and food, but over a lifetime, everyone is exposed to some methylmercury.

• **Ethylmercury** is formed when the body breaks down thimerosal. The body uses ethylmercury differently than methylmercury; ethylmercury is broken down and clears out of the blood more quickly. Low-level ethylmercury exposures from vaccines are very different from long-term methylmercury exposures, since the ethylmercury does not stay in the body.[19]

In the FDA's risk assessment, maximal potential exposure to mercury from vaccines was calculated for children at six months and two years old. The FDA used the US childhood immunization schedule to determine likely exposures. Those amounts were then compared with the limits for mercury exposure developed by the Environmental Protection Agency (EPA), the Agency for Toxic Substance and Disease Registry, the FDA and the World Health Organization (WHO).

The results of the risk assessment caused the medical community to make a change in the formula for childhood vaccines. "Depending on the immunization schedule, vaccine formulation and infant weight, cumulative exposure of infants to mercury from thimerosal during the first six months of life may exceed EPA guidelines."[20] Taken alone, that sentence sounds alarming, but it was then followed by this one: "Our review revealed no evidence of harm caused by doses of thimerosal in vaccines, except for local hypersensitivity reactions."[21] Nonetheless, the researchers said, you can essentially make the concern go away by simply using products formulated without thimerosal as a preservative.

So today, the only childhood vaccines that have trace amounts of thimerosal are one DTaP (diphtheria, tetanus and pertussis) vaccine and one DTaP-Hib (Haemophilus influenzae) combination vaccine. However, here is why some parents still get concerned about even trace amounts of the preservative: The standard immunization schedule calls for a child to get five shots of DTaP between birth and age six. Even though ethylmercury doesn't accumulate in the body, some parents have a concern about the repeated exposure, even to trace amounts.

The following paragraph from Robert Kennedy, Jr.'s white paper "Thimerosal: Let the Science Speak" (the source of material for his book of the same name) summarizes his views on the preservative and on media coverage of the supposed threat; the superscript numbers after the first sentence refer to a series of endnotes:

> Public statements have neither reflected nor acknowledged a vast, accumulating and compelling body of research that contradicts official safety contentions.[7][8][9][10][11][12] Evidence from epidemiological, animal, cell culture and clinical studies in the United States and from abroad suggests that the mercury in Thimerosal can cause brain injury in children.[22]

The endnotes are for articles in *The New York Times, Los Angeles Times, San Francisco Chronicle, USA Today* and *New Scientist.* For the record, all of the endnotes are links:

- Endnote 7 is represented by an article posted to the *New York Times* website on June 25, 2005, but following the link results in a "Page Not Found" error message. However, a search of the *New York Times* archives does yield an article on the same subject and published on the same day. Entitled "On Autism's Cause, It's Parents vs. Research," the article disagrees with both sides of the issue, first suggesting that a child might have too much mercury in his system from eating too much fish and, later, by rejecting the points made by the research team of Dr. Mark Geier and his son, David. One particular statement the article disagrees with is this: "Another study examined the records of 467,450 Danish children born from 1990 to 1996. It found that after 1992, when the country's only thimerosal-containing vaccine was replaced by one free of the preservative, autism rates rose rather than fell."[23] In interviews and writing, Kennedy has referenced Denmark as an important source of information on the purported link between autism and thimerosal, specifically because it is a country where autism rates could be examined in both "before" and "after" studies. Many feel the data indicates just the opposite of what Kennedy asserts.[24]

- Endnote 8 is an article in the *Los Angeles Times* reporting on the fact that the so-called vaccine court heard three cases and rejected the link between autism and mercury. Though Kennedy disagrees with the media who don't cover anti-thimerosal science, the following statement acknowledges that some kids are damaged by vaccines: "The court has made many awards to parents who successfully showed that their children were damaged neurologically or otherwise by vaccinations—a rare, but nonetheless real event—but has refused to accept claims that autism is caused by vaccination."[25]

- Endnotes 9 and 10 refer to news reports in *The New York Times* and *San Francisco Chronicle*, respectively, regarding studies in 2007 and 2008 that conclude there is no link between autism and thimerosal. Here is where Kennedy has an opportunity to make his case about a possible bias in the mainstream media or at least foreshadow the case to be made later: If there were studies published in the same timeframe that suggest a causative effect between thimerosal in vaccines and an increase in autism rates and these studies were ignored by the media, then these need to be included in order for the argument to have substance.

- Endnote 11 is about the swine flu vaccine and the article only makes a passing reference to thimerosal.

- Endnote 12 is an opinion piece written by an anthropologist for *New Scientist*; therefore, this article differs in intent from the other pieces, which are news items.

The one assertion from the Kennedy excerpt that really required endnotes is this: "Evidence from epidemiological, animal, cell culture and clinical studies in the United States and from abroad suggests that the mercury in Thimerosal can cause brain injury in children."[26] Precisely the same statement appears in the Executive Summary of Kennedy's book.

Here is how someone debating Kennedy on the issue of thimerosal might make the points that mirror his:

Public statements have reflected and acknowledged a vast, accumulating and compelling body of research that supports official safety contentions. Evidence from epidemiological, animal, cell culture and clinical studies in the United States and from abroad suggests that the mercury in thimerosal does not cause brain injury in children.

Endnotes supporting the first sentence could be the same as Kennedy's. Endnotes supporting the second assertion could refer to the following study, among others: "Thimerosal-containing vaccines and autistic spectrum disorder: a critical review of published original data" by S.K. Parker, B. Schwartz, J. Todd and L.K. Pickering, published in the September 2004 issue of *Pediatrics* (114(3):793–804).

In a debate with Robert F. Kennedy, Jr. on the issue of thimerosal, both parties would likely agree on one thing: Regardless of the cause, we as a society need to pay attention to the alarming rise in the rate of children diagnosed with autism spectrum disorder (ASD). One in sixty-eight children is a bad number, even if it includes a certain percentage of misdiagnosed cases.

CHAPTER 7

The Natural Immunity Debate

A mother brought her one-year-old baby to see coauthor Chris for a check-up. The baby had never received a single vaccination. The mother told Chris, "I see absolutely no reason to pump a healthy body full of chemicals. It's been proven that natural immunity is longer lasting than artificial immunity from a vaccine."

We have three comments about this mother's assertion:

1. The technical definition of natural immunity is an immunity that's present without immunization or sensitization. That means it's something children have before they're even born, because while fetuses are still in the womb, they are already acquiring antibodies from the mother.

2. Artificial immunity is one type of acquired immunity. It's the kind you get from vaccination or from an injection of immune globulin, which is used to treat a body with a weak immune system. The counterpart to artificial immunity is naturally acquired immunity. This results when antibodies

develop after exposure to a disease ("active immunity") or when antibodies are transmitted from mother to child though placenta or breast milk ("passive immunity"). With this clarification in mind, the name of this chapter really ought to be "The Naturally Acquired Immunity Debate," but that sounded a little too technical to us.

3. No, natural immunity is not necessarily longer lasting than artificial immunity from a vaccine. Let's refine this explanation by stating that the mother in the scenario was actually talking about naturally acquired immunity; depending on whether it was acquired actively through exposure to antigens or passively by transmission from the mother, the immunity may or may not last longer than what you get from a vaccine.

Our opinion: We see vaccines as providing "natural" immunity. The vaccine supplies the antigen before people are exposed to it in the environment, but the immunity that the body develops is real. It's as real and as natural as any other immunity your body generates.

Parents who believe it's better for a child to get a disease that probably isn't life threatening—and these typically include measles, mumps, chickenpox, flu, rotavirus and whooping cough—seem comfortable with ideas that don't make sense to most doctors. Exposing a child to these diseases is not just a matter of mortality, but a matter of morbidity; the disease is accompanied by symptoms that can be awful for a child. Secondly, in treating the disease after the child gets it, medications are generally involved. These can include antibiotics, cough medicine, anti-diarrheal medication and more. In the case of chickenpox, there may be permanent scarring.

Parents who choose not to have any care from the medical establishment are a different matter entirely. They fall into two camps, which are not mutually exclusive: people who have faith-based reasons for avoiding the medical establishment and people who are devoted naturopaths. People with faith-based reasons for avoiding all medical care unquestionably jeopardize their children if they are sick and the parents don't know what ailment they have. That's exactly what happened with Kara Neumann, whose juvenile diabetes was never diagnosed. Her parents' prayers for her health did nothing to stop her dying from diabetic ketoacidosis, which essentially makes it impossible for the body's organs and muscles to function.[1]

Naturopaths don't tend to be so absolute in their refusal to cooperate with the medical establishment. They espouse an alternative approach to medicine, refusing vaccines and even treatments such as chemotherapy, but they may well trust physicians who use naturopathy (or at least respect it) in the context of their regular practice.

SUPPORTING NATURAL IMMUNITY IN A BABY: HOW FAR DOES IT GO?

There are three key periods in a baby's life in terms of protective antibodies transferring from mother to child.

The first period is the last four weeks of pregnancy if the baby is full-term; premature babies get less of this protection. During that time, the flow of antibodies from mother to fetus via the placenta increases. This type of antibody is called immunoglobulin G (IgG). The immunoglobulins circulate in the blood and have an important role in disease protection up to about four months of age. Maternal antibodies passed on through the placenta are cleared by the infant around that time, which is why we see increased otitis media (ear infections) at that age, despite breastfeeding. Breastfeeding helps, but those placental antibodies work better.

The second period is during a vaginal birth, when the baby becomes coated with microbes from the mother's birth canal. These microbes contribute to gastrointestinal (GI) tract health and it appears they may have a protective effect in relation to certain health threats. They also colonize the baby's GI tract and remain there throughout his entire life. Babies born via C-section are not coated with these microbes—they acquire "hospital microbes" instead of "mommy microbes" in their GI tract.

However, new research published in 2014 examines one way to possibly rectify this problem. Maria Gloria Dominguez-Bello, an associate professor in the Human Microbiome Program at the New York University School of Medicine, has proposed using gauze to gather the mother's birth-canal bacteria and then swabbing the baby born by C-section. Her preliminary research indicates that this helps the baby's bacterial population to more closely resemble that of babies born vaginally.[2] C-section babies are at greater risk of developing asthma, allergies, obesity and other problems, so Dominguez-Bello analyzed ways to give those babies the same advantages as vaginal-birth ones. So far, she has only had partial success:

> When we analyzed the sharing—how many microbes any site of the baby's body share with their mom's vagina—we doubled the number of bacteria that the C-section babies were exposed to. But the vaginal process was six times as much. So the vaginal delivery still exposes the baby to a lot more.[3]

The third period is in the months or even years after birth when the baby is breastfed. Breast milk provides immunoglobulin A (IgA) antibodies, which help protect the baby from GI diseases such as diarrheal infections. A naturopathic mother's approach to sustaining natural immunity is to follow a long course of breast-feeding with a well-designed diet. And when the mother can't breastfeed, the recommendation in this community is to prepare a homemade formula to avoid the sugars, aluminum and geneti-cally modified ingredients found in pre-made versions.

Breastfeeding is highly recommended as long as the mother has a good nutritional program and a lifestyle and career that allow it. (Coauthor Maryann interviewed a chemist who was advised not to breastfeed because of the substances she was around every day.) The problem with homemade formula is that, like so many elements in a natural immunity program, some ingredients are hard to find and/or expensive. A one-month supply of ingredients costs about $200.

We interviewed one naturopathic mother who refused to get any vaccinations for her five-year-old son and one-year-old daugh-ter. She was emphatic that her son had never been to a doctor, because he had never even had a cold. He also never received any medications: "Not an aspirin or Tylenol or cough syrup—nothing!" The mother attributed much of her son's healthy condition to the fact that he had been breastfed for eighteen months. This is more than wishful thinking on her part: There are some very positive effects of breastfeeding that can last for several years. In one study published in the *Annals of Allergy, Asthma, and Immunology* journal, a Swedish researcher concluded that "There is also interesting evidence for an enhanced protection remaining for years after lactation against diarrhea, respiratory tract infec-tions, otitis media, Haemophilus influenzae type b infections and wheezing illness."[4]

But just because a protective effect lasts for a few years, that doesn't mean it will still be there when this little boy encoun-ters chickenpox at seven or eight years old—a distinct possibility since his mother indicated that, of the twenty-four kids in the neighborhood, six had not been vaccinated. A small percentage of vaccinated kids can also fall victim to chickenpox, although their case is often much milder, so the risk factors for unvaccinated kids are increased even further. The son may well have health advantages due to his nutrition and good genes, so maybe he will be more resilient than his peers when a disease strikes. That doesn't mean he will avoid disease, though.

NATURAL IMMUNITY LIFESTYLE
Lacey Grabel is the mother of two unvaccinated children: a three-year-old and an infant. The genesis of her concern about vaccination was learning that a dear friend's seemingly healthy two-month-old baby had had a seizure.

> Before I had kids, I had no interest in any of this stuff. Then a friend of mine had a son first and a little girl next. Two months after the daughter was born, she had a seizure. Then at six months, she had another seizure.
>
> [My friend's mother] asked, "Did the first seizure happen after she went to the pediatrician?" My friend went back to her baby book and was able to figure out that, yes, it happened the same night after [she] went to the pediatrician to get her [baby] shots. The same thing happened after the six-month appointment.
>
> She said that she was 100 percent convinced that it was the shots. And I thought, "How can that be?"
>
> That stayed with me.[5]

Lacey's three-year-old daughter is thriving, as is her young son. The daughter has never been sick and never received any medication. The advantages of natural immunity were created by a full-term pregnancy followed by a normal, vaginal birth and two years of breastfeeding. The lack of medication means that the child has not had microorganisms living throughout the body that perform vital functions in terms of overall health. Among other things, these microorganisms help prevent damaging, disease-causing bacteria from attacking the body and give advantages in absorbing and using nutrients in food.

Building natural immunity means, by necessity, avoiding "broad spectrum" antibiotics to whatever extent you can. Broad spectrum antibiotics are not targeted, meaning that many of them put a hole in the cell wall of certain good bacteria. Others starve the good bacteria by preventing protein synthesis. By "targeting specific bacteria," we mean that the antibiotic will work on the organism we think it will work on, but it will not kill everything else in the vicinity. For example, some antibiotics will kill both gram positive and gram negative bacteria. If we "target" a particular bug, we are only killing gram positive bacteria and leaving the gram negative bacteria alone. Another example is anti-viral medications like Acyclovir, which actually target Herpes viruses and leave your normal cells alone. We're not that good on specific bacteria just yet.

All communities should converge on the issue of antibiotics. The proper use of them does not have to do with vaccination directly, but it does become an indirect factor. Whether you choose to vaccinate or not, the resilience of your child's immune system is vital to fending off disease.

There is a correlation between people who gravitate toward natural/organic food stores and the percentage of the population that chooses not to vaccinate their children. It reflects what we call a "natural immunity lifestyle" that is typical of many residents in a place like Boulder, Colorado. In the city of Boulder, organic grocery stores outnumber conventional stores and the rate of unvaccinated children is 25.57 percent, according to research jointly conducted in 2015 by *The Denver Post* and ABC 7 News in Denver. (The two news organizations then created an interactive map to allow parents to click on their Denver-area school district to find out the percentage of unvaccinated children; they can also get specific information on each school in the district as well.)[6] The Boulder percentage far exceeds that of any other school district, with Adams County representing the other end of the spectrum: Only 4.44 percent of their school kids are unvaccinated. The median household income of Adams County is about half that of Boulder. This is significant because, outside of Amish communities, a natural immunity lifestyle tends to be quite expensive.

On the positive side, the health-related services and products in Boulder support a sophisticated approach to immune system health. The key word here is "system." Boulderites are doing more than just buying organic produce and vitamins for themselves and their kids to boost immune health. They also have access to healthcare professionals with expertise in integrative medicine, including integrative pharmaceuticals. Integrative medicine combines practices of conventional medicine with those of alternative medicine. You are much more likely to find a medical or dental school grad who also knows how to manage ayurvedic cleansing in Boulder than in most other cities in America.

There are strong beliefs in the community that reinforcing immune system health in this manner—on a daily basis—provides greater benefits and far lower risks than vaccines.

GENES AND IMMUNITY

Genes & Immunity is a journal devoted entirely to this topic. Many areas of research covered in the journal relate to what we have discussed in this book about the relative need for vaccines. Some people are simply tougher than others genetically when it comes to disease resistance. The influenza pandemic of 1918–1919 killed between twenty and forty million people—even more than the sixteen million people killed during World War I. Coauthor Maryann's great aunt was one of those who had the flu and beat it. She lived to be ninety-nine years old, still able to blow out the candles on her birthday cake. Since Maryann's great aunt lived in a very rural area when she had the flu, state-of-the-art medical care was remote. She survived because of home remedies and good genes.

A study that was published in a 2015 issue of *Genes & Immunity* focused on the possibility that some men have immunogenic factors which seem to lower their susceptibility to the HIV virus. The cohort study involved 151 Rwandans and 762 Zambians over a period of twelve years.[7] As the research continues, it could yield valuable information to further development of a DNA vaccine to prevent HIV.

The research conducted by scientists in this field also suggests why there might be enormous variances in the way that different children respond to the same vaccine. One study concluded: "The variation in antibody response to vaccination likely involves small contributions of numerous genetic variants."[8]

In chapter 10, we explore the connection between scientists' knowledge of genes and the application of that knowledge to create a new generation of vaccines.

THE CONTROVERSY OVER HERD IMMUNITY

The existence of herd immunity for a particular disease is often cited as one reason why it's okay that some children do not receive vaccinations, either because they can't for medical reasons or because their parents reject vaccination. Unfortunately, vaccine-induced herd immunity has its own set of challenges. Not only that, but it's simply not possible to achieve herd immunity with every infectious disease.

Herd immunity occurs when nearly 100 percent of a population can no longer contract a disease. The actual number is somewhere in the nineties and varies from about 90 to 95 percent, depending on the source of the estimate. When herd immunity is achieved through vaccination, depending on the disease, members of the population will need to receive booster shots in order to sustain herd immunity. Inactive vaccines like the pertussis and injected polio are two that require boosters. According to the ACIP schedule, children should receive a total of four doses of polio vaccine by the time they are six years old and a total of five doses of pertussis as part of the DTaP shot. Currently it's also recommended that adults get DTaP boosters, primarily to prevent adult transmission to infants.

Adults might be in the habit of bringing their kids in for wellness visits and booster shots, but it is far less likely they do the same for themselves. That reality needs to be factored in when estimating whether or not a community actually has herd immunity to a particular disease. As one mother we interviewed noted, parents who choose not to vaccinate their children might count the kids in the neighborhood and the kids at school who also aren't vaccinated. The parents who don't vaccinate talk to each other; they know who they are. This mother then calculated that there were enough vaccinated kids to ensure herd immunity in her community for the full range of vaccine-preventable diseases. Except that she never considered the parents, babysitters and visiting relatives who came into contact with the unvaccinated kids and had waning immunity to a handful of diseases.

Another issue is that it just isn't possible to achieve herd immunity with diseases that morph, like influenza. With smallpox, measles, polio, diphtheria and rubella, for example, we can go from herd immunity to eradicating them, because they have one antigenic type and aren't carried by animals or anything else. If we can get rid of the disease in the population, we can get rid of it in the wild. The reason flu vaccines change from year to year is because the flu itself changes from year to year.

The additional complication is that it's possible to carry certain communicable diseases and show no symptoms. You may think your child has no exposure to meningococcal disease, but the CDC estimates that 5 to 10 percent of adults are asymptomatic carriers. Assuming that your unvaccinated child is safe, because you don't see any evidence of the disease, does not mean that he or she isn't around someone who has it.

NATURAL IMMUNITY VERSUS VACCINATION

The debate here is whether it is better to vaccinate your child or forgo vaccination to focus on strengthening natural immunity. Based on our interviews, survey and literature searches—and they do not constitute what we would call "research"—we have concluded that parents who have a holistic approach to health are often the most adamant about avoiding vaccines. And that means *all* vaccines, at least in the early years. Not even Robert Sears' alternative schedule in *The Vaccine Book* is acceptable to them. The only caveat we heard repeated was something like, "If she wants to do volunteer work in Africa when she's in college, then we have to rethink whether she needs vaccinations." In other words, imminent danger in what they consider an alien environment might make vaccines "the lesser of two evils."

The arguments in this discussion are often heated and sharp. There is a perceived right and wrong and it would be very difficult, if not impossible, to reach a compromise. For that reason, we've decided to represent this debate in the form of "natural only" and "pro-vaccine" bullet points related to different topics.

TOPIC: TAKING THE PATH THAT AVOIDS SIDE EFFECTS

NATURAL ONLY
- Jenny McCarthy's autism organization, Generation Rescue, lists side effects for all of the vaccines given to children on the ACIP schedule and even sorts the vaccines by brand since they contain slightly different inactive ingredients. It's a convenient

compilation and, for the most part, simply reflects what the manufacturers' own literature says about possible side effects. Parents who fear serious side effects or fear that the emotional trauma of them will harm their child may decide to go a natural-only path. Alternatively, they may decide that the child would be able to cope with side effects better and not be as traumatized if the vaccinations were given when he or she is a little bigger and stronger.

- Side effects can be very serious, otherwise there would not be so many claims filed with the Office of Special Masters of the US Court of Federal Claims, more commonly known as the "Vaccine Court." According to the US Government Accountability Office, more than 9,800 claims have been filed with the National Vaccine Injury Compensation Program (VICP) since 1999; they then go to Vaccine Court to be adjudicated. Since 2006, about 80 percent of the compensated claims have been resolved through a negotiated settlement.[9]

PRO-VACCINE

- There is some risk of side effects and they tend to be the milder ones. Certainly, no one wants to see a baby cry, have a fever or vomit, but what would be even worse is to see a baby suffer the profound effects of a preventable disease. We need to keep perspective on this: Everything in life comes with the possibility of side effects.

- Research continues to improve vaccines, not only in terms of safety, but also effectiveness. FluMist is a relatively new vaccine that is delivered as a nasal spray—meaning it's painless. Studies have shown that it prevented about 50 percent more cases of flu than shots in young children. Side effects also tend to be quite mild, such as a low fever and runny nose for a brief period.

TOPIC: DELIBERATE EXPOSURE TO A DISEASE TO CREATE NATURAL IMMUNITY

NATURAL ONLY

- Healthy children could build up immunity to childhood diseases like measles by being exposed to the disease itself. One mother in Arlington, Virginia brought the unvaccinated children of her friends together for a "measles party" with an infected child. She and the other mothers agreed to expose these five children to the disease concurrently. That way, they would all miss school at the same time and then return when healthy to reduce the chance of getting anyone else sick. Some anti-vaxxers see "pox parties," which is the generic name for any parent-approved gathering with the aim of intentionally infecting kids, as a useful tool in building the strongest immunity possible in children.

- There is plenty of historical basis for this kind of action. Since the early 1900s, parents have used intentional, carefully monitored exposure of healthy children to diseases as a way of educating their immune systems. They don't view it as a capricious act on any level, but rather as a controlled process in which they will knowingly care for a child who has a particular illness. They are prepared to manage the outcome.

PRO-VACCINE

- There is a concept in law called reckless endangerment and it refers to engaging in conduct that creates "substantial risk" of physical harm to another person. There are people in the pro-vaccination community who think that a pox party constitutes reckless endangerment. They might also call it child abuse.

- "Yasuko Fukuda, a private practice doctor at San Francisco's California Pacific Medical Center and vice chair person for the

California chapter of the American Academy of Pediatrics... warns that parents intentionally exposing their kids put them at risk of respiratory issues that can lead to pneumonia, a swelling infection that can result in permanent brain damage and hearing loss and a fatal disease of the central nervous system that doesn't develop until seven to ten years after being infected with measles."[10]

- Pox parties do have a long—and ugly—tradition, with some in the early 1900s referred to as "measles teas." Mothers sipped tea while children played with pathogens. More recently, measles/mumps/rubella parties were prevalent in the 1950s and 1960s prior to the introduction of the MMR vaccine. After that, the parties where varicella was the guest of honor continued up until 1995 when the chickenpox vaccine was introduced in the United States. Now bring this into the twenty-first century. Science writer and parenting columnist Melinda Wenner Moyer posted this on slate.com: "A few weeks ago, I stumbled across the [online] group 'Chicken Pox Parties—New York Metro Area.' It has 143 members, all of whom, I'm guessing, are parents who have chosen not to vaccinate their kids against chickenpox and instead hope to build their kids' immunity the old-fashioned way, by directly exposing them to the germs of a pox-infected child. They are not alone: [The same website] has fourteen other chickenpox party groups organized by geographical region and if you can't get to one in person, you can always ask to be sent a lollipop with an infected child's spit on it."[11] This seems like a Dark Ages approach to protecting our children. According to the United States Postal Service, the act of knowingly sending a pathogen in the mail can be seen as an act of bioterrorism—a serious crime.

TOPIC: CHOOSING HEALTHY HABITS OVER CHEMICALS

NATURAL ONLY

- Blogger Shane Ellison calls himself "The People's Chemist" and makes some assertions that you will normally hear from people who have a disdain for vaccines. One of them is that it's actually improved hygiene, sanitation and nutrition—not vaccines—that have raised natural immunity for a great number of people, particularly those in developed countries. To support his assertion, he cites the scientific research that led to Bruce A. Beutler and Jules A. Hoffman winning a 2011 Nobel Prize for their work concerning the activation of innate immunity. The question these researchers answered is how specifically we defend ourselves against bacteria and other microorganisms. Beutler and Hoffmann discovered receptor proteins that can recognize invading microorganisms and activate innate immunity, the initial part of the body's immune response. Ellison states, "And all of this occurs without vaccination!"[12] It is the core of his argument that kids can build immunity naturally, rather than rely on "antiquated vaccine theory."

PRO-VACCINE

- If you share Ellison's point of view, then you see bitter irony in the fact that the work of Beutler and Hoffmann led to the production of new vaccines. They are actually two of the three scientists who shared the Nobel Prize for their discoveries in immunity that year. The third is Ralph Steinman, whose research focused on adaptive immunity, not innate. Their collective landmark findings helped improve vaccines aimed at infectious diseases and enabled the development of new cancer-fighting drugs.

- The argument that polio and other diseases were actually eradicated by better hygiene, sanitation and nutrition—and this is what Ellison unequivocally states—is far-fetched. In the course of twenty-five years, from 1954 to 1979, polio went from being a public health nightmare in the United States to yesterday's news. It's unlikely that occurred because we washed our hands, took out the garbage and drank orange juice. But there's more: Ellison also says that cases of polio increased due to vaccination. One of the mothers we interviewed who has chosen a "natural immunity lifestyle" made this exact claim as well.

As a footnote to the last discussion on the deliberate exposure of children to certain infectious diseases, one of the mothers we interviewed defended pox parties and stated, "People aren't going to die if they get the measles. This isn't 1920." We conducted a ten-question survey to find out how people around the country felt about certain ideas associated with vaccination and we used that statement to lead off the survey. The result: 27 percent agreed with her.

Science gives us certain answers that we may not like or agree with and dissenters will do everything possible to prove that those answers are flawed. In general, no amount of evidence or arguing will change the minds of those dissenters. It is personal experience that either reinforces their stance or brings them over to the other side.

CHAPTER 8

The Homeopathy Debate

Homeopathy was developed by the German physician Samuel Hahnemann (1755–1843). Ironically, homeopathy was the original immunotherapy, the theoretical model on which vaccination is based.[1]

> Excerpt from an article on homeoprophylaxis
> that later calls vaccines "poisonous."

Homeopathic medicine stimulates the body's own healing response to prevent or treat illness. Vaccination stimulates the body's production of antibodies to provide immunity against a disease. So why would homeopathic and conventional medicine be at odds?

Coauthor Chris tells patients who are curious about a homeopathic approach to medicine that one of the best homeopathic things they can do is vaccinate. Homeopathy schools have taught that giving the body a small quantity of what is bad for it leads to developing a tolerance or resistance to the substance. Allergy shots are true homeopathy and vaccines follow a similar concept.

The end result is the same but the process is different: With allergy shots, the aim is to get the immune system to ignore the offending agent; with vaccines, the goal is to get the body to attack it. There are homeopathic practitioners around the world who are also doctors. These people don't find it inconsistent at all to recommend both homeopathic formulas and vaccines to their patients; they aren't at war with the so-called medical establishment.

In the United States, people tend to categorize homeopathy as an alternative healthcare practice, whereas in Australia and the United Kingdom, many people feel homeopathy is "complementary medicine" rather than simply an alternative. Queen Elizabeth II's physician, Peter Fisher, is both a medical doctor and a practitioner of homeopathy. The Queen, who trusted in homeopathy before Fisher was even born, was very public about her older children being vaccinated when the polio vaccine was first introduced. But skeptics and homeopaths are often locked in combat.

Many people in the homeopathic community who reject vaccination describe a preventative program call *homeoprophylaxis*. We will focus on this program later in the chapter, but first, it's useful to have a shared understanding of how a leading skeptic and a key spokesman for homeopathy express their respective points of view. In this case, the skeptic illustrates what he sees as the fraud of homeopathy and the defender explains its efficacy.

We've staged this difference of opinion not so much as a debate but as a fight. That's certainly how it seems in the media.

SKEPTICS VERSUS DEFENDERS

James Randi is known as a legendary skeptic who has taken on homeopathy with drama and humor. If he were in a boxing ring squaring off with an opponent, that person could well be Dana Ullman, whom ABC News called "homeopathy's foremost spokesman."[2, 3]

Although the assumption might be that Andrew Weil, well known for his work in alternative medicine, would stand in Ullman's corner waiting to mop his brow, Weil doesn't gloss over the credibility issues faced by the homeopathic community. He provides a reasonable and even slightly critical introduction to this discussion:

> Homeopathy is among the most controversial of alternative medical therapies. Since homeopathic remedies are so dilute that, in many cases, not a single molecule of the active compound remains in the final preparation, many scientists believe therapeutic action is impossible. Others contend that all healing attributed to homeopathic preparations is either a placebo response or simply a misreading of normal healing that occurs with the passage of time. Double-blind studies involving homeopathic treatment have yielded variable, conflicting results.[4]

There are three key principles in homeopathy. The first is called "the law of similars" or "like cures like." The name *homeopathy* itself comes from two Greek words meaning "like" and "disease" or "suffering." A website called Homeopathy Plus uses the onion to explain this premise. Vapors from onions trigger a tearing response in most people and often a runny nose as well. So a person suffering from hay fever who has watery eyes and a runny nose would take a dose of Allium cepa—a homeopathic preparation of red onion.[5] This example illustrates a central idea in homeopathy: What the substance can produce in the healthy, it will treat in the unwell.

The second principle is the reason why devoted people of the homeopathic community go to practitioners rather than just buy off-the-shelf products; it's the principle of the single remedy. That means a single medicine should address all of the person's symptoms. On April 20, 2015, the day that the FDA launched a hearing to investigate homeopathy, NPR featured the contested practice in a story that began with a woman's trip to her practitioner's office, for complaints of chronic laryngitis and low energy. The doctor looked at her throat, listened to her lungs and asked her some seemingly unrelated questions, such as whether or not she had any weird cravings. She told him she was craving salty and spicy foods. With all of her symptoms in mind, including these cravings, the doctor consulted the The Homœopathic Pharmacopœia of the United States (HPUS), the official compendium for homeopathic medicines. The HPUS gave the doctor guidance for selecting pills to meet his patient's needs.[6]

The third principle, that of "minimum dose," has two components. One relates to how many doses are given to the patient and the other describes the composition of the medicine itself. The practitioner prescribes a small number of doses and adopts a wait-and-see approach before prescribing more or changing course. Matching the medicine to the individual's need is a vital element in homeopathy, so if the practitioner sees no improvement, a new formula is probably in order.

The second aspect of "minimum dose" involves dilution of the active ingredient. The medicine itself is so diluted that only a very tiny amount of the active ingredient remains—so tiny, it may even be undetectable. A well-known homeopathic remedy for the flu is Oscillococcinum, a product manufactured by Boiron. The active ingredient is listed as Anas Barbariae Hepatis et Cordis Extractum or extract of Muscovy duck heart and liver. That makes sense, since birds can carry the flu virus—especially waterfowl like ducks. This specific extract is diluted to 200C, a homeopathic designation meaning that it's one part extract to 200 parts of liquid, in this case ethanol. It's an infinitesimal amount of active ingredient.

Peter Fisher, Queen Elizabeth's physician, described the nature of dilution during a debate on the effectiveness of homeopathic practices: "The controversial part, of course, is the use of very high dilutions...dilutions beyond the point...where no molecule, no molecular trace of the original starting substance is present."[7] What Fisher referenced is something known to homeopaths as ultramolecular dilution. That is, once something has been diluted 1:10 twenty-four times, in all probability none of the original molecules remain. The theory is that this method works because the water or ethanol providing the dilution has "memory." It stores information relating to the active ingredient.

In his TED talk on "Homeopathy, quackery and fraud," James Randi ingests what is supposedly a fatal dose of homeopathic sleeping pills onstage. He swallows thirty-two caplets—the entire bottle—of Hyland's Calms Forté with a glass of water at the beginning of his talk. Toward the end of his seventeen minutes onstage, he tells the audience:

> I just ingested six and a half days worth of sleeping pills. That certainly is a fatal dose. It says right on the back here [holding the container in his hands], "In case of overdose, contact your poison control center immediately" and it gives an 800 number. Keep your seats! It's going to be okay! I don't really need it, because I've been doing this stunt for audiences all over the world for the past eight or ten years.[8]

Randi is not the only one who has tried to prove his point in this manner. In February 2011, other skeptics gathered for an anti-homeopathy conference and consumed entire bottles of remedies just like Randi.[9]

Rather than take Randi's jab at Calms Forté at face value, we decided to look at the formula for the product to see why the company includes warnings that actually advise the user to:

- Ask a doctor about using the product if pregnant or nursing.

- Consult a physician if symptoms persist for more than seven days or worsen.

- Keep the medication out of the hands of children.

- And finally, as Randi indicated in his talk, contact a poison control center in case of overdose.[10]

According to the manufacturer, Calms Forté sleeping pills contain passiflora, avena sativa, humulus lupulus and chamomilla as the main ingredients.

- Passiflora is more commonly known as passion flower and is used to induce sleep and relieve muscle spasms. It may even be used for anxiety disorders and upset stomach. When the passiflora extract is sold alone, the concentration is usually 1:1 or 1:3. In this sleeping aid formula, the same extract is in a 1:10 dilution—one milliliter of passiflora within ten milliliters of water or ethanol. Manufacturers of homeopathic products list the relationship as "1X" for a 1:10 relationship and "1C" for a 1:100 relationship.

- Avena sativa is oats, which is supposed to have a calming effect. The dilution is the same as passiflora.

- Humulus lupulus is hops, as in the substance used to make beer. The dilution is the same.

- Chamomilla is chamomile, commonly found in teas recommended before bedtime. The dilution here is 1:100.

- The other miscellaneous ingredients, when translated into English, are calcium phosphate, iron phosphate, potassium phosphate, sodium phosphate and magnesium phosphate. (Coauthor Chris notes that one potential hazard of too much phosphate is kidney stones, so perhaps the warnings regarding pregnant women and poison control are related to that and not the "active ingredients.")

As a homeopathic remedy, the Calms Forté formula defies logic. Homeopathy is based on the law of similars—"like cures like"—so a heavily diluted espresso would make more sense as a sleeping remedy than a product like Calms Forté. In fact, this is something that the Homeopathy Plus website expresses in a very specific manner, as part of its basic description of the law of similars:

> Coffee has a powerful effect on the body. The first time a person drinks a strong cup of coffee, they will experience one or more of the following symptoms: racing thoughts, palpitations, increased urine production, shaking hands, excitability and restlessness. If that person drinks it before bedtime, difficulty in sleeping can be added to the list.
>
> While coffee produces these symptoms in a healthy person, the Law of Similars dictates that it should be able to relieve similar symptoms in the unwell—and this is exactly what it does. [For] a child brought to a homeopath with hyperactivity, agitated thoughts and sweaty, trembling hands, a homeopathic preparation of coffee...would relieve and correct their symptoms.
>
> Another person seeking homeopathic treatment for insomnia caused by racing thoughts and the frequent need to urinate would also be prescribed [a coffee preparation]. Their racing thoughts and urine production would settle, allowing them to easily fall asleep. Once again, coffee can relieve in the unwell the very symptoms it produces in the healthy.[11]

To understand the sense of this, consider that Ritalin is a central nervous system stimulant. It is given to kids who have Attention Deficit Hyperactivity Disorder (ADHD) so they can focus and stop fidgeting. However, the drug has the opposite effect on people without the disorder.

Combining a few botanicals and significantly diluting them (as is the case with Calms Forté) is not homeopathic medicine. In principle, allergy shots are more homeopathic and so are vaccines. It could be argued that the sleeping pill demonstration used to debunk homeopathic remedies should really have a different target. Even so, Randi's stunt gains some credence from the issue of dilution and the fact that Calms Forté is described by the manufacturer as being homeopathically prepared.

With the skeptic having taken his jabs, now it's Dana Ullman's turn. In discussing the sense of homeopathy in contrast to conventional medicine, Ullman asserts that doctors tend to go after symptoms, whereas homeopaths view symptoms as defenses. For instance, if the oil light goes on in your car, the traditional doctor would fix it by disconnecting the light: "Double-blind and placebo control trials will show you that, when you do that, it cures the car—for the next five hundred feet or so."[12] A medical example he gives is a cold. In this scenario, the body creates mucus as a way of flushing out the material that's causing the illness. Typical cold medicine dries up the mucus membranes, depriving the body of doing the very thing it should be doing to cure the cold. Ullman says it's the difference between healing and suppression. Homeopathy intends to mimic the defense (symptom) as a way to stimulate healing.

We need to point out that Ullman's assertion is only somewhat true as it pertains to how the body heals and somewhat true as it pertains to cold medicine. The immune system with antibodies and macrophages cures the cold, not the nasal secretions. The virus is already in the body at that point and the nasal secretions will not solve the problem. The virus is not taking a surfing trip out of the body on a wave of snot. Much like homeopathic remedies, cold medicine has different formulas, so it's important to find the right one that matches the patient's specific needs. Cold medicines can also lighten symptoms so the person feels enough relief to start eating, sleeping and exercising again—all of which can help promote healing and the ability to return to work or play.

Ullman even compares homeopathic medicine to vaccines, just as coauthor Chris does, because they are also based on the law of similars. However, despite this comparison, he still criticizes vaccination (an example of that is referenced in the next section on homeopathic vaccines or homeoprophylaxis).

As for how homeopathic remedies work—which is the area of attack that James Randi focused on—Ullman explains that manufacturers start with pharmaceutical grade water, so it's already distilled twice. The water is then put into glass containers and shaken vigorously again and again. Metal isn't used because of the problem of leeching, but even glass is not completely inert, so the shaking will cause silica particles to enter the water—six parts per million. This shaking process creates very tiny bubbles that move to the wall of the glass and bring oxygen down into the water. The pressure in the water also increases with this repeated shaking. Ullman says it's been measured at 10,000 atmospheres, which means that whatever medicine is put into the water will be pushed into the teensy silica fragments very strongly.

But how is this very diluted formula able to have any effect on the body? Ullman explains that the body makes effective use of key substances in diluted form if it needs them:

> None of these homeopathic medicines will have any effect unless our body is hypersensitive and really needs it. Ultimately, in all of evolution, every animal on this planet, every plant will be hypersensitive to what it needs. A shark will be hypersensitive to blood. Think about the volume of water in the ocean and yet they can sense blood in the water at a distance.[13]

Ullman's reference to sharks is accurate; *National Geographic* states that great white sharks can sense even tiny amounts of blood in the water up to three miles away—but there's an important difference.[14] In the case of sharks, it's not because they need blood for their own vascular system; it's so they can eat the bleeding animal and ultimately survive. It gives them an advantage over other animals in the ocean. Again, it's not because they need the blood. The blood they take from other animals does not go directly into their vascular systems; it's digested and the nutrients are repurposed for whatever the body needs the calories and materials for. It could be blood, bone, fat, skin and so on.

So when *doesn't* a homeopathic remedy work? Ullman says simply: "When it's the wrong one." He likens it to putting a magnet near a piece of plastic; there is no affinity. But when there is hypersensitivity and the right medicine is used, then it works.

Realizing that we have tried to give space to the defense of homeopathy, we still have to conclude this subsection by noting that Ullman's reasoning takes a homeopath off the hook for anything that doesn't work, because according to his logic, the body didn't really need it.

HOMEOPATHIC VACCINES: HOMEOPROPHYLAXIS

Now comes the leap of faith, if you had not taken it before. Ullman's explanation of why homeopathic medicine can be an effective treatment seems consistent: The body has a need and that need creates hypersensitivity. When the body senses that what it needs is nearby, it takes advantage of it. Knowing this, how would a homeopathic formula work as a prophylactic since, at least in theory, it's administered while the body is healthy and not in need of the substance?

We posed this question to homeopaths who had posted articles about homeoprophylaxis online. The issue of hypersensitivity is apparently not at play here, which begs the question: How does something that reflects ultramolecular dilution work without the hypersensitivity that we allegedly have when we need a substance? Isn't this one of those magnet-near-plastic situations that Ullman described?

In theory, the efficacy all comes down to the fact that homeo-prophylaxis relies on *nosodes*. The basic definition of a nosode is no different from that of live virus vaccine, except for the first two words: *homeopathic remedy* created from some element of the disease itself, such as a discharge or diseased tissue.[15] But nos-odes have something special going for them—it's the quality that makes them work. The disease is diluted in such a way that it gets reduced to an energetic form:

> Nosodes emit the same frequency as the original disease agent. This frequency acts to stimulate general immune system func-tion. Taking a dose is like taking a tiny dose of the disease itself. Because the nosode is energetic, there is no actual dis-ease present; however, when introduced to the body, the body behaves as if it has the disease for a moment. This process is sufficient to educate the immune system about that particular disease.[16]

In more than one article or paper, this spurious logic is inter-twined with an assertion that it's good for kids to get a mild ver-sion of infectious diseases, because this not only educates the immune system in the short term, but also provides long-term benefits. And theoretically, children who had been given nosodes would only get a mild form of the disease, if they even get it at all, because they already have their defenses shored up. The following explanation of some key benefits to experiencing infectious dis-eases is from Diderik Finne, a Certified Classical Homeopath prac-ticing in New York:

> Immune system development is a life-long process, but the first two years of life are a critical period. Breastfeeding and

a healthy environment obviously play an important role, but Chinese medicine also underlines the infant's need to expel toxins acquired in the womb. These toxins are eliminated naturally by way of the skin eruptions associated with the traditional childhood diseases: measles, mumps, German measles and chickenpox.

A 1995 Swiss study looked at the possibility that childhood febrile infectious diseases provide a life-long benefit in the form of increased resistance to cancer. The study was designed as follows: all cancer patients seen by one of thirty-five participating Swiss physicians between June 1, 1993 and Jan. 31, 1994 were entered. For each patient, a control person of the same age and gender who did not have cancer was selected randomly from the patient list of the same doctor. A questionnaire was then sent to both cancer and non-cancer patients asking them, among other things, to list any febrile infectious childhood diseases they may have had. The purpose of the questionnaire was not disclosed either to patient or physician.

Result: a history of at least one infectious childhood disease reduced the risk of all types of cancer (except breast) by 10 to 30 percent. Chickenpox was the most effective in reducing risk.[17]

A translation of the first paragraph is this: Our immune system is stronger if we can expel toxins acquired in the womb and diseases that make us break out in ugly, itchy rashes or cause our glands to swell grotesquely are a really good way to do that. A question it raises is: What toxins? Yes, there are toxins in the womb as a result of a woman living her life in an environment with exhaust fumes, pesticides and bottom-feeding fish on the menu. But as soon as a baby is born, some of those same environmental toxins reach the baby without any help from the mother.

So how does a case of chickenpox get rid of only the ones that she gave him?

As for paragraph two, Finne fails to mention that the thirty-five Swiss physicians who participated in the study were anthroposophic doctors.[18] Anthroposophy is a philosophy, not a branch of medicine. In addition, the referenced paper called "Febrile infectious childhood diseases in the history of cancer patients and matched controls" was published in *Medical Hypotheses*, which is described by its publisher as "a forum for ideas in medicine and related biomedical sciences."[19] It is not peer-reviewed.

Finally, as for the health benefits of chickenpox, let's return to Dana Ullman, who shared a link to the following article in February 2013: "Shingles Goes Epidemic: Chicken Pox Vax to Blame."[20] Although the original article and Ullman's link have both been pulled, an article with the same name appears on another website. It features a direct accusation that the varicella vaccine is causing a shingles epidemic.[21] (This theory was later discredited by CDC research published in the *Annals of Internal Medicine*.)

In the world of homeopathy, it's clearly better to forego the varicella vaccine so you don't put grandma at risk for shingles and get chickenpox so you can reduce your chances of getting cancer.

Ullman has publicly stated that he is not against vaccines, but he doesn't think they are for everyone. Going back to chickenpox, he makes the same case as many others in the homeopathic community: "Some acute infections, such as chickenpox and measles, may actually be important for children to experience as a way to augment and strengthen their emerging immune and defense systems."[22] That might be acceptable if you could guarantee that the child wouldn't get something like measles until he was in the first grade. But the reality is that, from 2001–2013, 28 percent of children younger than five years old with measles had to be treated in the hospital. Babies with measles are in real danger of getting pneumonia, suffering brain damage or deafness and even dying.[23]

Though we have aimed for a fair debate in this book, the conflicting explanations as evidenced by the hypersensitivity/nosode debate, questionable studies and fuzzy assertions from within the homeopathic community itself have made us wonder why a parent would ever choose it instead of a conventional immunization program. The main reason we found is fear. This fear is not associated with the antigens in the vaccine, since homeopathic vaccines would naturally have to contain some of the disease in order to work. The fear is of the additives, preservatives and adjuvants in vaccines. In theory, homeoprophylaxis only consists of a very tiny amount of active ingredient, so you don't have to worry about very tiny amounts of aluminum or phenol.

CHAPTER 9

The Political Debate

Franklin Delano Roosevelt, thirty-second president of the United States, helped bring the country out of the Great Depression with a series of programs known as the New Deal. Roosevelt's programs involved federal assistance of one form or another to millions of Americans—and it greatly expanded the role that the US government plays in the lives of most citizens today. At the time, the New Deal prompted debate over how much responsibility a government should have for the security of its citizens.

For many years, the liberal view has been that the government has a substantial responsibility to protect the health, safety, property rights and even financial well-being of all citizens. In contrast, the conservative view is that the government shouldn't put its tentacles too deeply into the daily lives of its people, so the growing role of federal government in health care, for example, has been vigorously opposed.

Someone from another country or another planet who knew nothing more than that about partisan politics in America could easily make assumptions like these: Liberals would logically be in favor of mandatory vaccinations as a public health measure. Conservatives would logically fight them on the basis of such actions being an incursion into the private lives of citizens.

But pro-vaxxers and anti-vaxxers don't fall neatly into liberal and conservative camps. In fact, the mix of political liberals and conservatives in the anti-vaxxer camp is a fascinating collection of people who probably vote for different candidates in nearly every local and national election. The same could be said for pro-vaxxers as well.

LIBERALS AND THE ANTI-VACCINATION MOVEMENT

If we look at exemption rates in the various states and tie those states to the 2012 presidential election between President Barack Obama and Governor Mitt Romney, then liberals dominate in the anti-vax movement. Later in this chapter, however, it will be clear that this is only one criterion for determining the relationship between politics and anti-vaxxers.

According to the CDC, in 2012 at least 4 percent of the kindergarten population was exempted from vaccines in eleven different states. (The number of religious or philosophical exemptions far exceeded the number of medical exemptions.)[1] In terms of the presidential election, here is how each of those states voted:

Oregon (7.1 percent); Obama +12
Idaho (6.4 percent); Romney +32
Vermont (6.2 percent); Obama +36
Michigan (5.9 percent); Obama +9
Maine (5.5 percent); Obama +15
Alaska (5.3 percent); Romney +14
Arizona (4.9 percent); Romney +9
Wisconsin (4.9 percent); Obama +7
Washington (4.7 percent); Obama +15

Colorado (4.6 percent); Obama +5
Utah (4.4 percent); Romney +48

Note: Illinois did not report 2013–2014 data. However, according to the CDC's 2012–2013 report, Illinois had a vaccine exemption rate of 6.1 percent. (Its vote margin was **Obama +17**.*)*[2]

Therefore, through the filter of a presidential election between a liberal and a conservative, we see that four out of five of the most anti-vaccine states based on exemptions voted liberal. Keep in mind that there are many people who don't send their children to kindergarten—only fifteen states require it—so those kids who stay at home until first grade or later would not be counted among these "exemptions" if they weren't vaccinated.

As a corollary, Oregon's high vaccination exemption rate of 7.1 percent is consistent with the choice of its largest city, Portland, to ban fluoridation of the water supply. And Vermont, with its 6.2 percent exemption rate, is among the thirty-five states that do not mandate fluoridation. These are liberal strongholds that back up their philosophy of quality of life with votes that most of the nation would label "contrarian."

One regionalized study published in *Pediatrics*, the official journal of the AAP, wasn't looking for the political leanings of anti-vaxxers, but the results of the research strongly implied these affiliations.

The study concluded that "underimmunization and vaccine refusal cluster geographically."[3] The study population included 154,424 children living in thirteen Northern California counties and it identified five statistically significant "vaccine refusal clusters." What's striking about them is the relatively high median household income and education level of much of the population—a high percentage of bachelors and graduate degrees. What's also striking is that these clusters tended to be politically liberal areas like northern San Francisco and southern Marin County.[4]

Statistics on exemption rates and voting habits, however, do not address the motivation of liberal parents to reject vaccination. The "why" behind the decision of these California parents is broadly termed a "personal belief" exemption. It could include anything, from a distrust of pharmaceutical companies to a conviction that the Mothership will come for them before there is an epidemic. That's because the language of the Personal Beliefs Exemption to Required Immunization form—now part of California history—had simply stated, "I hereby request exemption of the student named above from the required immunizations checked below because such immunization is contrary to my beliefs."[5] Of the forty-eight states that give exemptions for people who have religious objections to vaccination, only nineteen allow the kind of philosophical objections that California used to allow.

Now invert the numbers, because the law has changed in California. As we were writing this section, a backlash occurred. On June 30, 2015, Governor Jerry Brown signed one of the strictest vaccination laws in the country. Starting on July 1, 2016, all children enrolled in any schools or daycares programs must be vaccinated against whooping cough, measles and other diseases, regardless of parents' religious and other personal beliefs. The sole exception is children with specific medical conditions—and only if they have a doctor's note. The only other states with such provisions are Mississippi and West Virginia.

With Brown's signature on the law, the Reed Union School Board in Marin County finally got its way. On February 10, 2015, a first-grade boy stood on a chair to reach the podium microphone and address the Board and assembled citizens of his community. He made a case for barring unvaccinated kids from school so that he could attend. The first grader's immune system had been compromised by leukemia and the treatments for the disease, so he can't be vaccinated; he has to rely on herd immunity. But the relatively high exemption rate in Marin blew a hole in the herd immunity argument that many parents had for letting their unvaccinated kids attend school alongside him. The school district's Board of Trustees thought this first grader had a solid point and voted to support the effort to kill the personal belief exemption throughout California. One of two key legislators who introduced the successful bill is a pediatrician named Richard Pan.

Because the concept of "personal belief" has taken so many forms in different states, many journalists and researchers have tried to illuminate the specific kinds of beliefs that anti-vaxxers hold. Staying focused on the liberal camp for the moment, consider the following reasoning that surfaced in an article in *Science* magazine.

Science, a publication of the American Association for the Advancement of Science, published a piece called "Why the 'Prius Driving, Composting' Set Fears Vaccines" in January 2011—four years before the outbreak of measles linked to Disneyland put the vaccination controversy in the headlines. In the article, *Science* reporter Greg Miller asked Seth Mnookin, author of *The Panic Virus: A True Story of Medicine, Science, and Fear*, a pointed question about the politics of anti-vaxxers: "There's a perception that vaccine refusal is especially common among affluent, well-educated, politically liberal parents—is there any truth to that?"[6]

Mnookin's response didn't answer the question directly, but he did say the decision not to vaccinate was linked to a sense of entitlement for many people. According to Mnookin, these parents felt they had a right to resist vaccinations for their kids, because they could rely on herd immunity. As noted in chapter 7, some scientists estimate the threshold for herd immunity to be about 95 percent; the CDC puts the vaccination rate for measles, mumps and rubella at only 91 percent.

Not giving up, Miller circled back to the core question: "But why liberals?"[7] Here was Mnookin's response:

> I think it taps into the organic natural movement in a lot of ways. I talked to a public health official and asked him what's the best way to anticipate where there might be higher than normal rates of vaccine noncompliance and he said take a map and put a pin wherever there's a [natural food store]. I sort of laughed and he said, "No, really, I'm not joking." It's those communities with the Prius-driving, composting, organic food-eating people.[8]

The public health official that Mnookin quoted gave a boots-on-the-ground assessment of the situation, but there are studies to back him up. Dr. Jennifer Reich, a sociologist at the University of Colorado Denver, has been researching the motivations of anti-vaxxers since 2007. In May 2014, she published a study called "Neoliberal Mothering and Vaccine Refusal: Imagined Gated Communities and the Privilege of Choice." Reich found that "parents who intentionally reject vaccines (versus undervaccinated children who may lack access to care or at least perceive that they do) look different. Children who are intentionally unvaccinated are more likely to be white, have a college-educated mother and a higher family income."[9] The conclusion she reached might be best summarized as follows:

> These parents shared a sense that avoiding infection was an individual responsibility, which could be successfully navigated via practices such as feeding their children organic food, monitoring who they spent time with and raising them to be responsible decision makers.[10]

Reich is very specific about her assessment that so-called neoliberal mothers who refuse to vaccinate their children feel that people who carry harmful, contagious diseases are simply outside of their network. Therefore, they see the entire process of protecting their children as manageable.[11]

One of the bridge reasons for rejecting vaccination—a reason that might be given by either a liberal or a conservative—is that it runs counter to religious beliefs. But it isn't the liberals who generally assert that they are the ones who personally hold those religious beliefs. Their contribution to the anti-vaccination movement is more likely to be found in showing support for overly broad religious freedom laws. Protecting the rights of Christian Scientists and some sectors of the Amish community may have been the original intent of exemptions based on religious grounds, but the protection of philosophical/conscientious objectors asserting any flavor of religious belief has grown well beyond that purpose.

CONSERVATIVES AND THE ANTI-VACCINATION MOVEMENT

A good place to start looking for anti-vaxxers among conservatives is in the "religious right." First of all, let's define the religious right as a movement that emerged in the 1970s in response to the Supreme Court's 1973 *Roe v. Wade* ruling which granted women the right to have an abortion and the "free love" mentality that swept through the nation at that time, particularly in many urban areas and on college campuses. The term "family values" is a keyword for this movement.

Because of their socially/sexually conservative positions, members of the religious right tend to oppose the human papillomavirus (HPV) vaccine. HPV is a group of more than 100 related viruses, some of which cause warts and others that can lead to cervical cancer. People get HPV through sexual contact with someone who has the virus. The problem some people have with the HPV vaccination is that the scheduled time to get it—and the ideal time in terms of the immune response—is in the pre-teen years.

For those of the religious right, adolescent sex is not compatible with "family values."

There is a politically conservative corollary to the religious argument about HPV vaccine that should be noted here. Some on the right see mandatory HPV vaccinations as "government intrusion into parental sovereignty."[12] It's an argument that could also support rejection of other vaccines administered to children.

The rubella vaccine in use today causes problems for many on the religious right for a reason that's related to the rejection of the HPV vaccine: It is essentially immoral. In this case, that's because the rubella vaccine had its origin in tissue from an aborted fetus. But the history behind it doesn't involve some mad scientist urging women to have abortions so he can experiment with disease prevention.

The rubella researcher Stanley Plotkin at the Wistar Institute in Philadelphia had access to an aborted fetus because, at the height of the rubella epidemic in the mid-1960s, many women terminated their pregnancies for fear that congenital rubella syndrome (CRS) had affected the fetus; the likely outcome could include cataracts, deafness, heart disease, encephalitis, mental retardation and pneumonia, among other serious health conditions. After one of the affected fetuses was sent to Plotkin's lab, he isolated the rubella virus and grew it in a cell strain developed by a Wistar colleague, Leonard Hayflick, whose source material was lung cells from an aborted fetus. The cell strain was free of contaminants, which were a concern related to vaccines made from animal material like duck embryo cells or dog kidney cells.[13]

Plotkin's vaccine was licensed in Europe in 1970 and nine years later in the United States. It replaced the rubella component in the MMR combination vaccine and has been in use ever since. Acceptance of the current rubella vaccine includes some traditionally conservative religious groups, such as the Roman Catholic Church. While the Church does urge its members to seek alternative vaccines to those made using the cells of aborted fetuses, it also says that "there is no moral obligation to use products that are less effective or inaccessible."[14] However, non-acceptance on the basis of the original reliance on tissue from aborted fetuses still prevails in certain conservative religious communities.

As for the other vaccines, there are some that were also developed with human strains similar to that of the rubella material, so these may be singled out as "unacceptable" to the religious right as well.

There are some religious people with an even more sweeping argument against vaccines. Anyone who takes the Old and/or New Testaments of the Bible literally might embrace a Bible-based argument against vaccination, summarized by this posting on the Vaccine Awareness of North Florida website:

> There are scriptural passages that teach us why it is not right to vaccinate. Vaccines are composed of foreign proteins and vaccination is the forcible procedure for putting foreign proteins in our bodies. Scripture gives specific instructions about how we are to care for our bodies and repeatedly warns against defiling the body. We are commanded to keep these temples clean, pure and holy.[15]

Religion is not the only basis for political conservatives to reject vaccination. For some, it is a matter of home rule—meaning, "I get to make the rules in my own home." Colorado provides a good example of this belief in action from a political standpoint. Despite the fact that Colorado law explicitly states that parents must vaccinate their kids or provide documentation of an exemption, the state appears to have the lowest vaccination rate in the entire country.

For the remote community of Gold Hill (population 230, according to the 2010 census), the exemption rate is 82 percent.

Gold Hill Elementary School is one of three schools in liberal Boulder County with an exemption rate of more than 50 percent and one of eight in the county with an exemption rate that tops 20 percent. But politicians and veterans of campaigns to vaccinate Colorado's children see the naturopathic parents of Boulder as an anomaly; statewide, they associate the refusal to vaccinate more with a pervasive limit-government-intrusion mentality, which they link to political conservatives.

Colorado and Utah have very similar laws, but Utah's vaccination rate for children in kindergarten is 98 percent, because Utah has enforcement provisions that Colorado does not. The political question is: Who is responsible for Colorado's practice of non-enforcement—left or right?

James Todd is a pediatrician who has been involved in a fight to vaccinate Colorado's children since 1971. As the director of epidemiology at Children's Hospital in Colorado, he is a logical spokesman for the pro-vax community. Todd's take on the reasons for non-enforcement of the vaccination law and the source behind that mindset is this:

> In Colorado, it's not a clinical issue. It's not scientific issue... Vaccinations have been a partisan, ideological issue that is not dealt with effectively.
>
> It's an opportunity for parties to highlight their philosophies and play to their bases...For the Democrats, it's been that vaccines work, are safe and we should require them. For Republicans, it's about personal freedom, parental choice.[16]

Todd's opinion is reinforced by the facts. First, state Senator Kevin Lundberg, a Replublication with children who are not fully vaccinated, fought a 2014 bill in the state legislature that would have made it harder for parents to forego vaccinations; many of

Lundberg's Republican colleagues sided with him and successfully defeated it.

After the defeat of that bill, Colorado Republicans introduced new legislation to give parents the right to make all medical decisions for their children. When this bill was first discussed in a hearing, anti-vaxxers of all stripes cheered together.[17] The "Parents' Bill of Rights" was approved on a party-line vote.

For some, an anti-vax stance represents an attitude toward science—a distrust and skepticism that may extend into many different branches. This is not the kind of counter to a scientific theory that involves a body of research. Instead, it is what researchers have called "conspiracist ideation," which "typically is not limited to individual theories, but represents a broader cognitive style or personality attribute."[18]

We labeled the liberal voters of Portland, Oregon—who made fluoridation of the water supply illegal—as contrarians. That's exactly the same term we would apply to the conservatives who reject science that they don't quite understand or find appealing. It's their "cognitive style" to doubt, in knee-jerk fashion, what government, mainstream science or others in a position to affect the entire populace assert as "good for you" or "widely accepted as fact."

That's not essentially a bad thing any more than it's a bad thing to question the free-market motives of pharmaceutical companies that make vaccines, as some liberals do. It's just a reminder of something that Gregory Hartley and coauthor Maryann suggested in *The Most Dangerous Business Book You'll Ever Read*: Extremes can mimic each other. In this example, the comparison being made is between individualists and collectivists, so the analysis is not politically oriented, but it does address the same personality types that are seen in this anti-vaxxer discussion:

On the healthy side, an individualist sees everyone's voice as vital. Every person should have the right to do and contribute as he pleases...Collectivists believe that looking out for the group's good is the most important action they can take and that individuals will find fulfillment in satisfying group needs...

On a radial scale moving from left to right, a collectivist can go so far left that he creates a culture that imposes one person's will on all others. By the same token, if an individualist goes too far in the opposite direction, he creates a culture in which the strongest of the group dominate and collectivism is inevitable. In this way the two extremes mimic each other.[19]

LIBERALS VERSUS CONSERVATIVES: THE HPV VACCINE DEBATE

When the focus remains on babies and children in the early school years, concerns about autism, the number of shots, corporate greed and related issues tend to take center stage for many parents who reject vaccination. They are joined—uncomfortably—by people whose religious or anti-government beliefs dismiss vaccines as "evil." These strange bedfellows sent the same message again in 2007 when the push first began to mandate vaccination of young girls against HPV with Gardasil—the one and only HPV vaccine at the time, which was manufactured by Merck. *The New York Times* reported:

> Groups wary of drug industry motives find themselves on the same side of the anti-vaccination debate with unexpected political allies: religious and cultural conservatives who oppose mandatory use of the vaccine because they say it would encourage sexual activity by young girls.[20]

The conversation shifted for both liberals and conservatives, though, sometimes pitting factions of them against one another. At other times they stood in the same corner, because distrust of Big Pharma and distrust of Big Government forced them to agree. Science generally crept into the discussions, but mostly the arguments were infused with politics.

The New York Times is considered to be one of the most important news sources for liberals, according to the Pew Research Center.[21] Nine days after reporting on uneasy alliances related to the HPV vaccine, they published an editorial entitled "A Necessary Vaccine." It stated: "State legislatures should require that all young girls be given this vaccine, which protects against a virus that causes some 10,000 new cases of cervical cancer in the United States each year—and 3,700 cancer deaths."[22]

With Merck initially lobbying hard for mandatory vaccination, one might have expected the pro-business *Wall Street Journal* to come out with a similar editorial. But it did not. *WSJ* instead declared: "Making Gardasil Vaccination Mandatory Would be Unwise, Academics Say." The post-comma phrase in this headline took *WSJ* off the hook in terms of sounding anti-business, but the sentiment was the same. The piece quoted experts making this key point: HPV vaccine doesn't address the same kind of threat to public health as measles or polio.[23] As a corollary, one of the experts added that including the HPV vaccine on the list of mandated immunizations would "exceed the original purpose of mandatory, school-based vaccinations."[24] This is an extension of the conservative argument that anything that inflates the size and authority of government is bad.

Thus, the liberal versus conservative debate on the HPV vaccine started to take shape. Five years later, *Forbes* directly stated that the conversation was political far more than it was scientific. This assertion emerged from a story about Neal Fowler, the CEO of a small biotech company. Fowler was diagnosed with a type of throat cancer that has now become quite common; it's a tonsil tumor caused by the same strain of HPV virus that causes cervical cancer. In the article, Fowler said that more patients like him would emerge unless something was done. He questioned why more young people are not immunized. Here is *Forbes'* analysis of that question:

> A big part of the answer is politics. Drug safety, vaccines, antibiotics and reproductive medicine—all have become proxies for the culture war, often tripping up public health in the process. Big Pharma hasn't helped, with deep P.R. wounds that have made it anathema to both political parties. Nor has the FDA, which has shifted the goalposts on approving new antibiotics enough to scare away many innovators just as resistant bacteria have become a big health problem. Both parties undermined the FDA further by overruling it on how the Plan B emergency contraceptive should be used, weakening the agency's authority. Now a coalition on the right is pushing to remove all testing of whether some medicines are effective, while many on the left still think the FDA remains too cozy with the drug industry.
>
> "If you look at both sides of the political spectrum I'm amazed and appalled by the lack of knowledge that's being put forward as knowledge," says Robert Ruffolo, former head of research at Wyeth. "They're not scientists, they're not physicians and many politicians will say almost anything during election season."[25]

Dan Kahan at Yale Law School perceived the political nature of the HPV vaccine debate very early on. He and a team that included colleagues from George Washington University Law School, Stanford University and the University of Washington designed a study called "Who Fears the HPV Vaccine, Who Doesn't, and Why?" One of the insights noted in the introduction to the study is this: "Although the public argument features competing empirical claims, the battle lines are decidedly political."[26] Our connection to groups that we feel are integral to our personal identity has a huge influence on our views, such as what we fear or what we determine is a low-risk threat. Main groups for many people are race, gender, religious affiliation and political party membership.

We can understand how liberals and conservatives differ on the issue of HPV vaccination if we consider that the two groups have certain competing values which shape conflicting views on what is good or not good for society. What are the societal risks and benefits of certain actions? Each side believes that if the country went in its direction and not the other way, we would all be better off. "Premarital sex must be discouraged" is a value statement that criticizes anything that makes premarital sex safer, because if it's safer, then it's more desirable. "Teenage curiosity about sex is normal and healthy" is a value statement that criticizes efforts to make it harder to have safe sex. Each side believes society will be better off if their point of view is supported through laws and regulations—or the lack of laws and regulations.

Kahan and his team found two mechanisms in play that profoundly affected their stance on the public health consequences of mandatory HPV vaccination: biased assimilation of information and source credibility. "Biased assimilation refers to the tendency of individuals selectively to credit and dismiss information in a manner that confirms their prior beliefs."[27]

Source credibility involves not only a person's perception of the knowledge and honesty of the source, but also a sense of affinity to the source itself. If your parish priest comments that mandatory HPV vaccination is a flawed idea, but a Nobel Prize

winner in medicine who is an atheist says that it's vital, the Nobel
Prize might not be a persuasive credential.

The risk-benefit perception statements presented to the
1,538 participants in Kahan's study were as follows:

POLICYNEED. It is important to devise public health
  policies to reduce the spread of HPV. [Strongly disagree,
  disagree, agree, strongly agree]

HPVSAFE. The HPV vaccine is safe for use among young
  girls. [Strongly disagree, disagree, agree, strongly agree]

VACDANGER. Universal vaccination of girls for HPV will
  likely endanger their health. [Strongly disagree, disagree,
  agree, strongly agree]

HPVACTIVE. Universal vaccination of girls for HPV will
  lead girls to become more sexually active. [Strongly
  disagree, disagree, agree, strongly agree]

FALSESECURITY. Girls vaccinated against HPV are more
  likely to engage in sex without a condom. [Strongly
  disagree, disagree, agree, strongly agree]

HPVBENEFIT. How beneficial would you say universal
  vaccination of girls against HPV is likely to be? [Not at
  all beneficial, slightly beneficial, moderately beneficial,
  very beneficial]

HPVRISK. How risky would you say universal vaccination
  of girls against HPV is likely to be? [Not at all risky,
  slightly risky, moderately risky, very risky][28]

The study participants were divided into three groups. All
three were presented with an introductory note that simply said
some public health experts are in favor of mandatory HPV vaccination and others are against it. After reading the note, the first

group responded to the statements with no further explanation provided; this was called the "no argument" group. The second group received brief "for" and "against" arguments, just like the ones you would see on a ballot to explain the reasoning behind initiatives up for a vote; this was the "unattributed arguments" group. The third group responded to the statements after exposure to "culturally identifiable advocates." These participants read what opposing experts had to say about the issue and were told that each one was on the faculty of a major university and had written books on public policy. They were shown photos of the four experts along with the names of their books.

What the third group of 1,022 participants didn't know was that the experts were entirely fictional. The photos showed two white men in business suits, one white man with a more avant-garde look and one white man with a casual, open-collar shirt and a beard. They represented what anthropologist Mary Douglas described in her work sorting people according to "group" and "grid:"

- High group people put the needs of the community over those of the individual; they are called "communitarian."

- Low group people are "individualistic;" people should take care of themselves without interference from the community.

- High grid people see the world in a "hierarchical" way; there's a stratification based on certain characteristics.

- Low grid people eschew that stratification and support an "egalitarian" social order. [29]

The white guys in suits were both hierarchical, with one leaning toward individualistic and one leaning toward communitarian. The avant-garde man and bearded man were both egalitarian, with the avant-garde man being on the individualist side and the bearded man communitarian.

At the outset, the study designers predicted that the most extreme differences would be between the hierarchical individualist and the egalitarian communitarian. To suggest the kind of profession each might have—not the kind of character—the designers labeled one the founder and CEO of a company and the other a social worker. The result based on their data was this:

> ...The types of subjects we predicted would be most disposed to react in extreme ways to arguments—increases from .16 in the "no argument" condition to .57 in the "unattributed arguments" condition or .41 overall, a statistically significant change.[30]

Fitting into the hierarchical/individualist quadrant meant the person was far more likely to have grave concerns about the risks of HPV vaccination than those in the egalitarian/communitarian quadrant. We'll come right out and state the obvious: The hierarchical/individualist is most likely a political conservative and the egalitarian/communitarian is most likely a liberal. In an expression of the "digging in your heels" response when a belief is threatened, "the size of the disagreement between subjects with those values grew when they were exposed to balanced arguments."[31]

Kahan and his colleagues wondered if there might be any way to achieve a convergence of views. Is it possible to at least minimize the polarization?

This is what we've tried to do in this book. Our method seems to be consistent with Kahan's, even though we had no knowledge of his study when we first began this effort. He has proposed a "pluralistic argument environment." It's a scenario in which people are exposed to experts with diverse values on both sides of the debate.

CHAPTER 10

The Future of Vaccination Debates

Vaccine research responds to public health crises, from the Ebola epidemic in West Africa to the global HIV/AIDS pandemic. If many scientists are talking about an "epidemic" or "pandemic," then chances are good that someone, somewhere is taking action to create a vaccine to combat it. The same can be said for serious, chronic illnesses like tuberculosis, cancer and Alzheimer's disease. According to the Pharmaceutical Research and Manufacturers of America (PhRMA), nearly 300 vaccines to prevent or treat such diseases were in development as of 2015. These vaccines include:

- A genetically-modified vaccine for the treatment of pancreatic cancer
- A therapeutic vaccine that increases the immune response against the HIV virus
- A vaccine that protects infants against meningococcal disease, a leading cause of meningitis
- An immunotherapeutic vaccine for the treatment of Alzheimer's disease
- A recombinant vaccine to prevent malaria[1]

Many people who have been affected by these diseases desperately want the vaccines to become available. However, the vaccines still have to go through a number of developmental stages first. The CDC lists them as:

- Exploratory stage
- Pre-clinical stage
- Clinical development
- Regulatory review and approval
- Manufacturing
- Quality control[2]

Clinical development is a three-phase process. In Phase I of vaccine trials, small groups of people receive the vaccine to test its safety. In Phase II, the vaccine is given to people who are intended to benefit from the immunization and the overall number of recipients is expanded. In Phase III, the question to be answered is: Does the vaccine work with a large number of those targeted to receive it?

The stages of the vaccine development cycle are not likely to change, but we can see at least three things that are changing now and will continue to evolve in relation to the emergence of vaccines:

- How vaccines are developed
- What health threats vaccines will protect against or treat, including non-infectious conditions such as Alzheimer's disease and drug addictions
- Methods of administering vaccines

These areas of progress reflect the development of what might be called "vaccine technology." Even most vaccine skeptics today should be able to embrace the concept of progress in this context. What the vaccine contains, how it works, who needs it or doesn't need it, what eliminates or minimizes trauma from vaccination—these are all issues guiding current research. It's research that will deliver the next generation of vaccines.

We can also project with certainty a change in human beings that will affect how we view and use vaccines: The day appears to be coming when genetic manipulation could negate the need for vaccines as we know them. The aim of vaccines is to make us stronger and better able to fend off threats to our health. The aim of naturopathic or homeopathic medicine is arguably the same, as is a type of genetic manipulation called *genome editing*. But in regard to the latter, there is another important dimension of genome editing technology: the hope of curing diseases that we now consider incurable.

MANUFACTURING THE NEXT GENERATION OF VACCINES

Molecular biology has changed the possibilities for making vaccines. Stanley Plotkin, a physician who helped develop the rubella vaccine, has stated that the new technologies allow scientists to create nearly any antigen they want, or really any substance that could be useful in vaccination, in the laboratory.[3] To understand what these new manufacturing possibilities give us in terms of safety and efficacy—and why some of the techniques may change a lot of minds about vaccination—it's useful to have a little background on how the process first started and how it has developed until now.

We've come a long way since May 14, 1796, the day that Edward Jenner first tested his smallpox vaccine. His healthy patient was an eight-year-old boy named James Phipps. Jenner began by scratching fluid from a cowpox blister into the boy's skin; only one blister rose up in response. Jenner then repeated the process using smallpox material; the boy never caught smallpox. Jenner's vaccine was a live virus that had been **attenuated**, meaning it was weakened to the point where it should have been safe. The vaccine could trigger an immune response, but it wasn't strong enough to bring about a full-blown case of the disease.

Live, attenuated vaccines have never been effective for everyone. People who have a compromised immune system from disease or chemotherapy typically should not be given live vaccines. At the same time, this form of vaccination does a great job of educating a normal immune system so it learns to fight a disease naturally; this is something that homeopaths and naturopaths would agree with in principle. The downside is that live viruses and bacteria still have the potential to cause the disease the vaccine is trying to prevent. This is one reason why scientists have looked for other ways to make effective formulas to counter the same illnesses. Another downside is that these vaccines need refrigeration or else they will spoil.

The live, attenuated vaccines made out of viruses (as opposed to bacteria) are generally easy to make. One popular way to attenuate a virus involves growing it in a hostile environment. The virus has to fight for its life and that struggle effectively weakens it. As the virus evolves, attempting to adapt to the alien environment and survive, it loses the ability to do serious damage to its natural host—a human being.

Kids still receive live, attenuated vaccines to prevent the following diseases:

- Measles
- Mumps
- Rubella
- Flu (only if they get the nasal spray called FluMist)
- Chickenpox
- Rotavirus

- Polio (only the oral version, which is not the one commonly given to kids in the United States and is currently being phased out worldwide)

The common version of the polio vaccine now given is an **inactivated vaccine**. In this case, the disease-causing microbe is killed by chemicals like formaldehyde, radiation or heat. Inactivated vaccines are more stable and considered safer than any formula containing a live virus. Because the active ingredient is dead, the immune system's response is weaker than it would be with live, attenuated viruses or bacteria; the use of an adjuvant like aluminum is therefore more important with an inactivated vaccine than with a live one. Booster shots are also common with this form of vaccination. Kids receive inactivated vaccines to prevent the following diseases:

- Polio
- Pertussis

A third, more sophisticated manufacturing process produces **subunit vaccines**. The premise is that subunit vaccines don't contain the entire microbe, but instead have just the antigens that do the best job of stimulating the immune system. In some cases, it isn't even the whole antigen, but a piece of it. The first step is identifying which antigens or parts of the antigens are needed to combat the disease. Step two involves growing the microbe in a laboratory and then using chemicals to break it apart. An alternative second step is to manufacture the antigen molecules using recombinant DNA technology, essentially joining segments of DNA together. Because subunit vaccines contain the most important antigens and parts of antigens and no other molecules that compose the microbe, the chance of having a bad reaction to them is diminished. Kids receive subunit vaccines to protect against the following disease:

- Hepatitis B

The manufacturing process changes according to the cause of the disease. In the case of illnesses resulting from a toxin released by the virus or bacteria, the vaccine is made of the deactivated toxin (or toxoid) rather than the whole virus or bacterium. To deactivate the toxin, the sample is treated with formalin, a solution of formaldehyde and sterilized water. Kids receive **toxoid vaccines** for the following diseases:

- Diphtheria
- Tetanus

A **conjugate vaccine** emerges from a process that's designed to help infants get more benefits from vaccination. This is how the National Institute of Allergy and Infectious Diseases explains the way that conjugate vaccines are manufactured:

> If a bacterium possesses an outer coating of sugar molecules called polysaccharides, as many harmful bacteria do, researchers may try making a conjugate vaccine for it. Polysaccharide coatings disguise a bacterium's antigens so that the immature immune systems of infants and younger children can't recognize or respond to them. Conjugate vaccines, a special type of subunit vaccine, get around this problem.
>
> When making a conjugate vaccine, scientists link antigens or toxoids from a microbe that an infant's immune system can recognize to the polysaccharides. The linkage helps the

immature immune system react to polysaccharide coatings and defend against the disease-causing bacterium.[4]

Young children receive a conjugate vaccine for the following disease:

- Haemophilus influenzae type B (Hib)

We began the modern-day process of vaccine development by taking a smear of actual disease. Next we moved on to reducing the amount and using treatment to weaken it, before inactivating it whenever possible. After that, we relied on increasingly smaller bits of the illness-causing substance as the active ingredient. A **DNA vaccine** is the next logical step in this evolution: It gets right down to the microbe's genetic material. In this new experimental process, scientists aim for the genetic code of the antigens. With DNA vaccines, we are officially entering "the future."

Researchers have found that the genes of a microbe's antigens get a strong response from a human being's antibodies, as well as a strong cellular response. The body is ready for combat on multiple levels. Administering the vaccine might be through a traditional injection technique or by using a high-pressure gas or nasal drops.[5] This technology is explained a little more in the following section on new ways of administering vaccines.

Comparatively speaking, a DNA vaccine is a "cheap vaccine," because DNA is stable and easy to manufacture. It's also a reliably "safe vaccine," since it can't cause the disease when there's no microbe present. Researchers just haven't arrived at the point yet where these vaccines are as dependable as desired in terms of eliciting an immune response. DNA vaccines are being tested right now in the fight against viruses that cause influenza and herpes, among others. They also offer hope of immunizing against parasitic diseases like malaria. Here is an overview of the advantages and disadvantages of DNA vaccines:

ADVANTAGES OF DNA VACCINES

- Inexpensive
- Long-term persistence of immunogenicity, the ability to provide an immune response
- Subunit vaccination with no risk for infection
- Ease of development and production
- Immune response focused only on the antigen of interest
- Stability of vaccine for storage and shipping
- DNA vaccines are safer, more stable and easy to handle
- DNA vaccines induce protective humoral (associated with circulating antibodies) as well as cellular immune responses
- DNA vaccines are heat stable
- A mixture of plasmids (genetic structures in cells) could be used to form a broad spectrum vaccine

DISADVANTAGES OF DNA VACCINES

- Limited to protein immunogens (not useful for non-protein based antigens such as bacterial polysaccharides)
- Certain vaccines, such as those for pneumococcal and meningococcal infections, use protective polysaccharide antigens
- Inducing antibody production against DNA
- DNA vaccines may have a relatively poor immunogenicity
- Atypical processing of bacterial and parasite proteins
- Insertion of foreign DNA into the host genome may cause the cell to become cancerous[6]

The list of disadvantages makes it clear that the future of these vaccines is not a perfect scenario. Nonetheless, optimism surrounds the current development of DNA vaccines to prevent or treat a number of diseases, such as:

- **Cancer**—The vaccines aimed at countering cancer fall into both the prophylactic and therapeutic categories; discussions of vaccines to prevent breast cancer and to treat pancreatic cancer appear later in this section.
- **Tuberculosis** (TB)—The vaccine is designed to treat TB.
- **Edwardsiella Tarda**—This is a nasty bacterium that can affect humans, animals and fish. It not only causes gastroenteritis, but is also a culprit in septicemia, meningitis and wound infections. The vaccine aims to trigger a protective autoimmune response.
- **Human Immunodeficiency Virus** (HIV)—This cause of AIDS remains a global killer; the vaccine designed to combat it is a DNA vaccine in the "recombinant vector" category.
- **Anthrax**—Primarily associated in the western world with bio-terrorism, anthrax is a zoonotic disease, meaning it can be transmitted from animals to people. The vaccine would protect against it.
- **Influenza**—Just as there are many strains of the flu virus, there are many vaccines in development to prevent them.
- **Malaria**—With about half of the world's population at risk of malaria, there is aggressive investment of financial and human resources to develop vaccines that both treat and protect against it.[7]
- **Dengue**—Like malaria, the source of this fever is mosquitoes and the vaccine in development aims to protect against it.
- **Typhoid**—A salmonella bacterium causes typhoid fever and the fight to prevent contraction has involved both live, attenuated as well as DNA vaccines that are currently in clinical trials.[8]

DNA research has also led to another experimental form of immunization called ***recombinant vector vaccines***. These vaccines are made through a process that might seem dated at first glance: It involves a weakened virus or bacterium, but the difference between recombinant vector vaccines and older vaccines of this nature is how they get the job done:

> [Recombinant vector vaccines] use an attenuated virus or bacterium to introduce microbial DNA to cells of the body. "Vector" refers to the virus or bacterium used as the carrier.
>
> In nature, viruses latch on to cells and inject their genetic material into them. In the lab, scientists have taken advantage of this process. They have figured out how to take the roomy genomes of certain harmless or attenuated viruses and insert portions of the genetic material from other microbes into them. The carrier viruses then ferry that microbial DNA to cells. Recombinant vector vaccines closely mimic a natural infection and therefore do a good job of stimulating the immune system.[9]

Recombinant vector vaccines offer hope of replacing our current immunization for rabies and measles with something that's both effective and involves fewer risks. They also serve as a model for experimental HIV vaccines.

FUTURE PROTECTION

Returning to Plotkin's focus on how molecular biology is providing scientists with new tools, he notes that we aren't just talking about diseases caused by infectious agents anymore when it comes to vaccines. In a broader way, he states "We can determine which substances within microorganisms are important in causing disease and therefore which ones we should choose to use to try to prevent the disease from occurring."[10]

Plotkin is not only referring just to contagious diseases like measles, but also to chronic diseases like cancer, Alzheimer's and diabetes. In his estimation, fighting them with vaccines is becoming more realistic. This is a provocative proposition, but not without ramifications in the marketplace that could affect whether or not the vaccine is made available to the public in a timely manner.

Just about anyone can contract an infectious disease if exposed to it. Unless there are people with Superman genes when it comes to measles or the flu, we are all susceptible. Immunization is what the majority of people in places like the United States have sought to become more like Superman. The market for those vaccines is huge and insurance companies acknowledge that vaccination is an anticipated expense for the majority of families. Even in the face of high costs of clinical trials, companies have a strong economic incentive to develop vaccines for the masses.

One of the relatively new vaccines in this category is the HPV vaccine, designed to prevent contraction of types 16 and 18 HPV, which are responsible for causing about 70 percent of all cases of cervical cancer worldwide.[11] Another one, Gardasil, is also approved to prevent vaginal and vulvar cancers in females. The only other FDA-approved preventative vaccine for cancer is one that protects against Hepatitis B infection, so it averts the development of liver cancer related to Hep B.

Other cancer prevention vaccines that don't involve an infectious disease are on the horizon as well. For example, a vaccine to prevent breast cancer has been pioneered by Vincent Tuohy at the Cleveland Clinic, perennially one of the premier health facilities in the United States. This vaccine targets a protein found in breast tumors, but generally not in healthy tissue. Tuohy explains, "We've reasoned that if we immunize against this protein that the normal tissue wouldn't be affected but the emerging breast tumors wouldn't occur. They would be destroyed as they emerge."[12] In his paper on the effort, published in the April 27, 2010, issue of *Nature Medicine*, Touhy explains how the vaccine has proven effective in studies with mice.[13]

Touhy's vaccine would be a single-shot solution to the most insidious type of breast cancer called "triple-negative breast cancer," the form most often seen in women with BRCA1 (breast cancer susceptibility gene 1) mutations. Awareness of BRCA1 and BRCA2 shot up when actress/director Angelina Jolie announced that she had undergone a preventative double-mastectomy after learning she had the BRCA1 mutation. Roughly half of the women with one of these mutations develop breast cancer by age seventy and the chances of inheriting it from a parent who carries the mutation are also 50 percent.[14]

In September 2013, after three years of effort to fund the breast cancer vaccine research, Cleveland Clinic Innovations was able to launch a company called Shield Biotech to develop Touhy's vaccine and take it through clinical trials. At the time of the announcement, their projected timeline for availability was ten years. That seems like a long time, considering that about one in eight (12 percent of) women in the United States will develop invasive breast cancer during their lifetimes, according to the American Cancer Society.[15]

As noted earlier in this chapter, there are six stages in the process of getting a vaccine from concept to public availability. With Touhy's vaccine, the estimated time to complete pre-clinical studies and get permission from the FDA to test it was two years. Shield Biotech estimated that it would take another three years to get through Phase I clinical trials. The dosage and safety tests would involve recovering women with triple-negative breast cancer and healthy women at high risk who chose to have a bilateral mastectomy as a preventative measure. The other five years in that ten-year estimate are consumed by Phase II and Phase III trials.[16]

Unless you have gone through the simple but not necessarily inexpensive process of genetic testing, you don't know if you are predisposed to cancer or if you carry genes that make your progeny, siblings and cousins predisposed to it as well. With the cooperation of insurance companies, that kind of testing could become routine, but it currently is not. So this begs the question: Would something like the Touhy vaccine move through trials more quickly if routine genetic tests confirmed that a high percentage of women have the BRCA1 gene? Nearly a quarter of a million women are diagnosed with breast cancer each year; the cost savings—which can hit $100,000 per patient for surgery, chemotherapy and radiation—would seem to justify the support for a faster track.

On the therapeutic vaccine front, there is also hope for people who already have cancer. However, as with the preventative vaccines, the process from initial development to clinical trials to availability tends to be very long. This is an especially painful reality for people with pancreatic cancer, when 80 percent of patients who undergo surgery end up relapsing and dying from the disease within five years.[17] As relatively rare as it is—approximately 1.5 percent of men and women will receive this diagnosis versus the 12 percent of women who will get breast cancer—it has caused the death of some of society's most famous names. Among them are tech innovator Steve Jobs, actor Patrick Swayze, Carnegie Mellon professor Randy Pausch (*The Last Lecture*) and opera tenor Luciano Pavarotti. Even when a disease has a famous face, however, there is no guarantee that the prevention or treatment of it will receive the funding and logistical support needed to swiftly move forward.

Researchers at Johns Hopkins University's Sidney Kimmel Comprehensive Cancer Center brought a pancreatic cancer vaccine to clinical trials in 2008, more than a decade after it was first developed. *Medical News Today* described it as a way to "reprogram" cancer tumors:

The vaccine, called GVAX, was developed by Johns Hopkins researcher Dr. Elizabeth Jaffee to "reprogram" tumors to include immune system T cells that are able to fight cancer. To accomplish this, GVAX is made of irradiated tumor cells that have been modified to recruit immune cells to the patient's tumor.[18]

The patients who participated in Jaffee's study underwent surgery to remove their tumors two weeks after they received the vaccine. The results held tremendous promise: The vaccine caused the creation of certain structures called "aggregates" in thirty-three of the thirty-nine patients who remained disease free. These structures helped to regulate immune cell activation. In other words, the tumors "learned" to combat the cancer.

Jaffee appeared on the *Dr. Oz* television show to discuss her work, immediately after which the Johns Hopkins clinic received more than one thousand inquiries from patients all over the United States. On an ongoing basis, the clinic gets an average of two calls a day from people who see hope—maybe their best hope—in the one vaccine that has been developed to help cure pancreatic cancer.[19] It's safe to say these people would probably pay anything to get their hands on it.

The same can be said for individuals and families affected by Alzheimer's disease, which the Alzheimer's Association notes is "the only cause of death in the top ten in America that cannot be prevented, cured or slowed."[20] With more than five million people in the United States afflicted with Alzheimer's, the annual cost to the nation is astronomical—an estimated $226 billion in 2015, according to the Association.

Unfortunately, news on the vaccine front has been disappointing. Since 2000, there have been a number of clinical trials for Alzheimer's immunotherapy, but they have all failed. There is still a bright side, however. The hypothesis as to why these trials haven't been considered successful is that the bio-markers of Alzheimer's precede the clinical symptoms by about twenty years and the immunotherapy to address it needs to begin before those symptoms surface. According to the coauthors of the study "Advances in the Development of Vaccines for Alzheimer's Disease," published in *Discovery Medicine* in 2013, "Treatment was started too late and too little."[21] So with that theory helping to shape new research, three trials have been launched to investigate when the therapy should really start. One of them is called the Dominantly Inherited Alzheimer Network (DIAN) study, which will focus on patients who are carriers of genetic mutations predisposing them to Alzheimer's.[22]

In contrast to a target population that has insurance coverage and/or other resources to pay the potentially high price of receiving a new vaccine, many populations afflicted with epidemics, pandemics or chronic disease need generous subsidies for inoculations. This is why it's difficult to bring a "benevolent" vaccine to market.

Sanofi Pasteur has been participating in a worldwide effort to create an HIV/AIDS vaccine for decades. People in many parts of the world experience HIV as a family health issue. In the United States, there is both a high-risk population, as well as many who probably would not get the vaccine—nor would insurance companies likely pay for it—because they are not at risk. Children and adults might be exposed to the seasonal flu or to whooping cough from the kids around them, but unless they are in certain health-care situations or having unprotected sex, they're most likely safe from HIV. So how much money would the company make on its HIV vaccine in the United States unless it charged a lot to offset the cost of basically giving it away in countries with HIV epidemics? These are the reasonable economic issues we have to confront when we demand excellent preventative medicine.

The issue of cost-effectiveness takes center stage in discussions of vaccines emerging to combat the Ebola hemorrhagic virus and drug addictions. Containing the Ebola virus, which killed nearly 11,000 people in 2014–2015, poses enormous challenges and the costs of meeting them are astronomical. The fight against Ebola involves the same three-pronged attack that's seen with any other infectious disease: education on how the virus spreads, identification of the natural reservoir host and vaccination. The challenges are interlaced.

The 2014 outbreak in West Africa triggered the largest Ebola epidemic in history. Not understanding how the virus spread from person to person, many people contracted the disease by caring for the sick and burying their dead. This direct contact with an infected person's body fluids exposed them immediately. An added challenge to educating the high-risk populations in this epidemic was the fact that a great many had no access to mass media technologies like the internet and television.

Despite the assertions of some scientists who are convinced the natural reservoir hosts of Ebola are bats, there is evidence to suggest that while bats might be carriers, they aren't the host species. We are certain of the hosts for diseases such as measles (human beings) and rabies (terrestrial mammals such as raccoons, skunks, foxes and coyotes, as well as several species of bats) and that knowledge greatly helps to contain them. Likewise, identifying the reservoir host of Ebola is "essential to preventing future outbreaks," according to all of the key scientists tackling the problem.[23]

One of those scientists is Eric Leroy, a French virologist who works in Gabon on the west coast of Central Africa. He describes the difficulty with identifying a reservoir host as threefold. First, the amount of virus in a host tends to be very low—much lower than in an infected person or animal. Second, the virus may have a low prevalence in a population—the percentage of those that test positive for infection may be small. So if the researcher trying to identify the host thinks the culprit might be one of three different kinds of bats, four different kinds of spiders or eight different kinds of insects, consider how many bats and spiders and bugs he might have to test until he finds one that has a detectable amount of virus in it!

> If a single kind of animal amid the great diversity of tropical forests represents a needle in a haystack, then one infected individual within one population of animals amid such diversity represents one needle in ten thousand haystacks.[24]

Understandably, the third difficulty in identifying the reservoir host is the cost. Field operations for this kind of endeavor are extremely expensive. This is partly because there is a possibility that the prevalence of the disease in the host may vary considerably based on the season. Therefore, studies would likely need to be ongoing, year-round, until there is a definitive identification of the host.

Without knowing where the virus comes from, the best hope that medical professionals have of combating it is with a vaccine. Fortunately, the virus seems to have "genome stability," meaning that it hasn't changed much since first being identified four decades before the 2014 outbreak.[25] This makes it quite different from HIV, for example, which mutates rather quickly.

As of this writing, only one Ebola vaccine, rVSV-ZEBOV, has made it to a Phase III efficacy trial. This vaccine is a product of research conducted by the National Microbiology Laboratory, a division of the Public Health Agency of Canada, which is like the CDC in the United States. And even though the trip from Phase I to Phase III for the rVSV-ZEBOV Ebola vaccine was less than a year—lightspeed compared to most vaccines—the efficacy trial was fraught with complications.

This timeline reflected the acute sense of governments and medical scientists that Ebola had emerged as a major public health crisis. The paper about the initial safety trial, entitled "Phase 1 Trials of rVSV Ebola Vaccine in Africa and Europe—Preliminary Report" was coauthored by fifty-eight contributors from various countries and published in *The New England Journal of Medicine* on April 1, 2015. Twenty-eight contributors coauthored the Phase III report, published just four months later on August 3, 2015, in *The Lancet*. This report was titled "Efficacy and effectiveness of an rVSV-vectored vaccine expressing Ebola surface glycoprotein: interim results from the Guinea ring vaccination cluster-randomised trial." The reference to "ring vaccination" means that the contacts of a person infected by Ebola—and those who had come into contact with those contacts—were vaccinated to determine if the vaccine acted fast enough to avert the spread of disease in that community.

Another kind of trial that is essential to having a firm grasp on the vaccine's efficacy is being conducted in Sierra Leone. This one aims to determine if the rVSV-ZEBOV vaccine can offer long-term protection against infection for people like healthcare workers. It is a joint effort of the CDC, the College of Medicine and Allied Health Sciences, University of Sierra Leone (COMAHS) and the Sierra Leone Ministry of Health and Sanitation (MoHS). Launched in April 2015—the same month the paper on the Phase I trial came out—the project is called the Sierra Leone Trial to Introduce a Vaccine against Ebola (STRIVE).

The raw numbers on the Guinea trial were outstanding: No one in the trial got Ebola. Taken at face value, the vaccine could be described as being 100 percent effective and that's exactly what some media outlets reported. But this high score looks far less believable when other data enters the picture.

The researchers targeted 4,123 people to get the vaccine as soon as possible due to their potential exposure. Of that number, 2,109 didn't receive it because they were too young, breastfeeding or unwilling to participate in the trial. Therefore, a little fewer than half—2,014—got the vaccine. Within the unvaccinated group, only eight contracted Ebola.

So is it more accurate to say that the vaccine prevented approximately eight cases of Ebola—an infection rate of 2.6 percent in the unvaccinated group—or that it's 100 percent effective because none of the vaccinated individuals got sick? Before regulatory bodies approve the vaccine for widespread use, they will have to make a determination such as this.

It's reasonable to wonder why there aren't more options for Ebola vaccines, considering the magnitude of the public health crisis in Africa. The explanation is partly hidden in the phrase "in Africa." In the case of Ebola, the target population cannot help defray the extremely high cost of developing the vaccine.

This high cost starts with the type of facility required to produce the vaccine. Developing an Ebola vaccine requires a Biosafety Level 4 (BSL-4) laboratory, which offers the highest standard of contaminant protection. There are only about two dozen of these facilities worldwide, compared to thousands of BSL-3 labs. The lone privately-owned lab of this caliber in the United States is located at the Texas Biomedical Research Institute and funded by a combination of government and corporate grants and contracts, as well as private donations. The other BSL-4 labs are affiliated with government or academic institutions. The University of Texas Medical Branch manages one of the few in the United States and lists the construction cost as $15.5 million.[26] Yearly costs of running and maintaining a lab like this are roughly double that amount and involve scores of doctoral-level scientists.

These construction costs almost sound inexpensive when the features of the lab are considered—and all of them are essential to protect researchers from Ebola and to protect the rest of us from such viruses escaping the facility. First of all, the lab has to be completely isolated from all other areas of the building or be in a separate building. Researchers work in a sealed shell that is both animal and insect proof, with specialized ventilation and exhaust components. In addition:

> The Biosafety Level 4 laboratory has special engineering and design features to prevent microorganisms from being disseminated into the environment. Personnel enter and leave the facility only through the clothing change and shower rooms and shower each time they leave... Personal clothing is removed in the outer clothing change room and kept there. A specially designed suit area may be provided in the facility...The exhaust air from the suit area is filtered by two sets of HEPA [High-efficiency particulate arresting] filters installed in series. Supplies and materials needed in the facility are brought in by way of double-doored autoclave, fumigation chamber or airlock, which is appropriately decontaminated between each use.[27]

Ebola vaccine isn't the only one that has very little appeal to developers when the cost of producing it can't be easily justified by the prospect of insurance company reimbursements down the road. For example, Kim Janda of the Scripps Research Institute, which is headquartered in San Diego, California, has made significant progress in the development of vaccines for heroin, cocaine and methamphetamine addictions. The most promising is the heroin vaccine, which went through preclinical trials in 2013.

The subjects of these trials were heroin-addicted rats and none of them relapsed after receiving the vaccine. *TIME Magazine* reported:

> Janda's vaccine works a bit like a sponge in the bloodstream. If a person—or in this case, rat—is inoculated, that "sponge" sucks up the drug and prevents it from reaching the brain. Some drugs for addiction will block receptors in the brain so when a drug reaches the brain it can't activate it like it used to; the heroin vaccine prevents the drug from reaching the brain at all.[28]

George Koob, director of the National Institute on Alcohol Abuse and Alcoholism, gave his assessment of the trials and their promising successes: "You can inject a rat with ten times the dose of heroin that a normal rat [could handle] and they just look at you like nothing happened. It's extraordinary."[29]

Yet despite these encouraging results, Janda cannot secure funding to go any further, because "no pharmaceutical company is going to fund trials for heroin."[30] This is just another way of saying that insurance companies aren't going to fund addiction vaccines even though the estimated annual healthcare cost related to tobacco, alcohol and illicit drug addiction in the United States alone totals $166 billion.[31] Ironically, these companies are picking up some of that cost through coverage of addiction treatment, which is mandated by forty-three of the fifty states, as well as the District of Columbia.[32]

WAYS OF ADMINISTERING VACCINES

Injections are old technology. Many of the science-fiction doctors we see in movies and on TV never poke anyone with a long needle. Instead they use something called a jet injector, which involves gently touching the patient and injecting a remedial substance with a "whooshing" sound. We can do this now and we aren't even living in the twenty-fourth century. Our twenty-first century version of that device has various names like Jet Injector Gun, Ped-O-Jet, Biojector 2000 and PharmaJet Needle-Free Injector. They are all designed to immunize without a needle by pushing the vaccine through the skin. For example, DNA vaccines can be administered with a needle and syringe or with a device that uses high-pressure gas to shoot microscopic gold particles coated with DNA directly into our cells.[33]

Applying vaccines to the skin without injecting them is one of the important new vaccination methods that vaccine pioneer Stanley Plotkin talks about in "The Future of Immunization."[34] He specifically references the fact that needles tend to frighten people.

FluMist is a flu vaccine that's administered as a nasal mist and has been shown to be highly effective among children. The rotavirus vaccine is given to babies orally in drops. If we do move to a point where the health benefits of vaccines are accepted by the majority of the population throughout life, not just in the pediatric age group, we will have to move toward some of the models seen in our favorite sci-fi movies. Too many people just don't like needles.

GENOME EDITING: THE FUTURE VACCINE?

During an April 28, 2015, discussion on NPR's *On Point*, titled "Re-Engineering Human Embryos," Nobel Prize winner Craig Mello said that genome editing might be used like a vaccine one day. The similarity is that the genetic change would be used to prevent a terrible disease; the difference is that it would only need to be done once and, theoretically, it would be 100 percent effective.

The human genome is constantly modified through mutation. And most of the time those [mutations] are silent or
even deleterious. If we have a way of improving and repairing
and making genes better, safer, healthier…You know, someday, it may be like vaccination where, if you have a child,
you'll want to have these [genetic] tests done and perhaps
have a correction made.[35]

This kind of genetic tinkering has been the subject of hypotheses and discussions ever since James Watson and Francis Crick
discovered the double helix structure of DNA in the 1950s.
However, some very controversial research heated up the conversation in 2015. An announcement by Beijing Genomics Institute
(BGI) about their work in gene editing suddenly brought the concept of genetically-modified people from science-fiction movies to
the attention of *The New York Times*. BGI scientists took a technique that was developed in the United States in 2012 and used
it on human embryos.

This process involves a relatively simple technology called
CRISPR (clustered regularly interspaced short palindromic
repeat). Carl Zimmer, science writer and columnist at *The New
York Times*, puts it in plain words:

Scientists discovered that bacteria were making some very
interesting molecules that could zero in on the genes of viruses
that were invading them. They would grab on to a particular
spot in the DNA and cut it. So these scientists said, "Wait a
minute. If these bacteria have evolved to zero in on a particular
spot of DNA and cut, we could use that as a tool."[36]

The scientists concluded they could target a piece of DNA that had
a defect, cut it out and insert a replacement segment of DNA that
did not have the defect. For example, there are ongoing clinical

trials which use a version of this process to prevent human cells from being infected with HIV; the same technology could also be used to effect a cure for patients with HIV.

The value of this work in terms of human health is to potentially avert all kinds of diseases. If the editing is performed on an adult, then it only applies to that individual, just like a vaccine. If it's performed on an embryo that's later implanted and born, however, the altered genetic trait becomes heritable. So an embryo that has had the BRCA1 gene altered to avert breast and ovarian cancer could produce offspring with the same protection against those cancers. Ethicists seem to think this is a very bad idea, because the changes to an embryo, sperm or egg will affect future generations. That could have strange consequences, since we don't really know what multiple jobs a gene might perform in the body. We are dealing with a system, not just isolated pieces and parts.

The international consensus among scientists is to keep the focus on preventing and curing disease for those already born.

IS THERE REALLY A DEBATE HERE?

Whether you feel your identity in this conversation is anti-vaxxer, pro-vaxxer, naturopath, homeopath, Big Pharma fan, public health official or bewildered parent, the future could bring us all together in some very critical ways. Only anti-science proponents would likely mock the attempts being made to make safer, more effective and even more customized vaccines.

Sometimes, these vaccines may even emerge as an unintended consequence of ongoing research to relieve the pain and suffering of sick patients. One example is a vaccine to protect against Group A streptococcus (GAS), which is a significant cause of infectious disease worldwide—GAS causes severe problems for about eighteen million people annually, with 500,000 of them dying.[37] On August 11, 2015, a simple article titled "Strep's evolution may provide clues for developing a vaccine" appeared in selected newspapers. It announced some hope for a way to combat Group A strep:

> The same bacteria that cause simple strep throat sometimes trigger bloodstream or even flesh-eating infections instead and over the years dangerous cases have increased. Now, researchers have uncovered how some strains of this bug evolved to become more aggressive.
>
> The bacterial sleuthing may offer clues for developing a vaccine against group A streptococcus.[38]

How could this be construed as anything but good news?

The common ground is that we don't want our children to be sick, nor do we want to be sick ourselves. And we don't want to put our children or ourselves at risk while we try to protect them.

Making Up Your Mind to Be Pro- or Anti-Vaccine

Imagine for a moment that we live in a world where the medical and pharmaceutical communities have addressed all concerns about the contents of and schedules for vaccines. Would a wave of parents suddenly flood pediatricians' offices and beg for the new, "safe" vaccines?

Based on history, that's highly unlikely.

On September 28, 2011, Professor Gareth Williams of Gresham College in London gave a lecture called "From Jenner to Wakefield: The long shadow of the anti-vaccination movement." Williams is the author of *Angel of Death: The Story of Smallpox* and a consummate storyteller whose lecture about the anti-vaccination movement illustrates how the same kinds of biases and fears have affected the adoption of vaccinations for centuries. Improvement of vaccines occurred steadily, but at no time did "everyone" get behind them and uniformly choose vaccination—even in the face of severe financial penalty and possible imprisonment in nine-teenth century England.

The tactics have not changed, either. Principal among them have been the use of anecdotes, getting celebrities to act as spokespersons, bending statistics to support a certain point of view and outright lying.[1] Does this mean that the pro-vaccination movement hasn't used the same tactics—at least occasionally? No. The techniques to propagate and sustain biases and fears—emotion-based factors in decision-making—haven't changed because they work. We have seen a repeated use of tactics that effectively sway public opinion and we are likely to see the same ones in use again tomorrow.

The over-arching reason for this is because there's a strong emotional attachment to personal points of view, whether sparked by anecdotes, information delivered by a celebrity, statistics or studies like that of Andrew Wakefield's "proving" a connection between MMR vaccine and autism (later proven to be false).

Remember that ultimately the argument both for and against vaccines is one of fear, the fear of what might happen. The difference is one of education and study. Franklin Delano Roosevelt got it right in his first inaugural address when he said: "The only thing we have to fear is fear itself."

The prime argument *against* vaccination plays on parents' fears that their child will have some chronic developmental damage and not be normal due to the vaccines. The argument *for* vaccination is based on the fear of infectious diseases that we have seen cause either death or severe, chronic developmental and neurological damage to children and adults around the world. We see that devastation of health and life as being preventable.

We hope you have found this book helpful in your search for fair, reasonable and science-based information about vaccines. *The Vaccination Debate* is intended as a path to well-informed conversations about whether or not to vaccinate your child.

Acknowledgments

We appreciate the tremendous support we've received from New Horizon Press: Dr. Joan Dunphy, Joe Jasko, JoAnne Thomas and Charley Nasta. Your encouragement and attention to detail make authors feel respected and valued.

Thank you to Lacey Grabel for her intelligent and candid contributions and to Laurie Watkins for helping us connect with Lacey. We also appreciate the many parents who contributed their experiences, insights and opinions anonymously. Whether you were sharing a fear or a hope, we heard the commitment to the well-being of your children in your voices.

Glossary

Adjuvant—an agent that may stimulate the immune system and increase the response to the specific agent in the vaccine; allows for dramatic reduction in the amount of antigen in the vaccine

Anthrax—a serious infectious disease caused by bacteria found in soil; anthrax is a zoonotic disease, meaning it can be transmitted from animals to people

Artificial immunity—one type of acquired immunity, specifically the kind you get from vaccination or by getting an injection of immune globulin

Autism—refers to a range of neurodevelopment disorders, also known as Autism Spectrum Disorder

BRCA1 and **BRCA2**—refers to Breast Cancer susceptibility gene 1 and gene 2 mutations, which predispose a person to breast and potentially other "female" cancers

Carrier species—a species that can transmit a disease from the reservoir host to another species, for example, human beings (see also, Reservoir host)

Case series—the type of study Andrew Wakefield used for his discredited research targeting MMR vaccine as a cause of autism

Chickenpox (varicella)—an infectious disease caused by the varicella-zoster virus which results in an itchy rash and red spots or blisters

Cohort study—one type of observational study involving groups of people that share common characteristics

Conjugate vaccine—a vaccine made by attaching an antigen to a carrier protein as a way to help trigger an immune response in a baby whose immature immune system wouldn't respond to harmful bacteria coated in sugar molecules (polysaccharides)

Diphtheria—an infection that causes a thick covering in the back of the throat that can lead to breathing problems, paralysis, heart failure and death

DNA vaccine—an experimental vaccine utilizing the genetic code for antigens

Double-blind study—neither the subjects participating in the study nor the research team know who receives the real medication and who receives the placebo

DTaP—a combined vaccine for diphtheria, tetanus and pertussis

Edwardsiella tarda—a dangerous bacterium that can affect humans, animals and fish; it causes gastroenteritis and has a probable role in septicemia, meningitis and wound infections

Epidemic—the rapid spread of an infectious disease (see also, Pandemic)

Formaldehyde—used in the manufacture of vaccines to inactivate viruses so that they don't cause disease; also serves to detoxify bacterial toxins, such as the toxin used to make diphtheria vaccine

German measles (rubella)—an infectious disease caused by the rubella virus; also known as the three-day measles

Guillain-Barré Syndrome—rare disorder in which the body's immune system attacks the nerves; often cited as a possible outcome of vaccination

H1N1—a type of flu virus that reached pandemic levels in 2009; also known as swine flu

Haemophilus influenzae B (Hib)—a bacteria family potentially resulting in severe meningitis, causing shock, sepsis (bacteria in the blood) and death

Hepatitis A—a liver infection transmitted via fecal matter

Hepatitis B—a liver infection often transmitted sexually, but can also be transmitted by contact with infected blood or other body fluids

Herd immunity—a concept which suggests that, once a certain percentage of a population has immunity from a disease, then the rest of that population is protected from the disease

Homeopathy—an alternative medical practice based on the notion that the body can be helped in healing itself through remedies that adhere to a "like cures like" approach

Homeoprophylaxis—homeopathic vaccine

Human papillomavirus (HPV)—a group of viruses, some of which can cause cervical, throat and other cancers

Humoral response—associated with circulating antibodies (as opposed to a cellular response)

Immunogenicity—the ability to provide an immune response

Immunoglobulin A (IgA)—antibodies transmitted in breast milk that help protect the baby from GI diseases such as diarrheal infections.

Immunoglobulin G (IgG)—antibodies passed through the placenta to the baby; they circulate in the baby's blood and have an important role in protection against disease up to about four months of age

Inactivated vaccine—a vaccine in which the disease-causing microbe is killed by chemicals like formaldehyde, radiation or heat

Influenza (flu)—an infectious disease caused by a number of different viruses that result in respiratory problems; not to be confused with what is called "stomach flu"

Intussusception—an intestinal disorder that causes a serious blockage; although it is uncommon for people of all age groups, it is more common in young children than adults

Law of Similars—a core principle of homeopathy, also represented as "like cures like"

Live, attenuated vaccine—a vaccine containing a live virus that has been weakened to the point of being safe; it can trigger an immune response, but isn't strong enough to bring about a full-blown case of the disease

Measles (rubeola)—a highly contagious respiratory disease characterized by a blotchy rash

Meningococcal disease—a quickly moving infection that can cause death within hours

MMR—a combined vaccination for measles/mumps/rubella

Mumps—an infectious disease caused by a virus that mostly affects the salivary glands just below and in front of the ears; the disease causes swelling in those glands

Natural immunity—immunity that is present without immunization or sensitization

Naturally acquired immunity—immunity that results when antibodies develop after exposure to a disease ("active immunity") or when antibodies are transmitted from mother to child though placenta or breast milk ("passive immunity")

Nosode—homeopathic remedy created from some element of the disease itself, such as a discharge or diseased tissue

Notifiable diseases—diseases that must be reported to government authorities

Oncogenic—describes something that causes tumors

Pandemic—large global outbreak of a disease

Pertussis (whooping cough)—an infection that can cause coughing spells so bad it's hard for the infant to eat, drink or even breathe

Phase I clinical trial—small groups of people receive the vaccine to test its safety

Phase II clinical trial—see Phase I clinical trial; this phase expands the trial, with the vaccine given to people who have similar characteristics to the target population for the vaccine

Phase III clinical trial—see Phases I and II; this phase involves administering the vaccine to thousands of people and testing to ensure that it is effective as intended

Plasmids—certain genetic structures in cells

Pneumococcal disease—a leading cause of serious illness throughout the world resulting from bacteria called pneumococcus, which has the ability to attack different parts of the body and cause ear infections, pneumonias, sinusitis, sepsis (a bloodstream infection), shock and meningitis

Poliovirus (polio)—a virus that can cause acute paralysis and often permanent physical disability and death

Recombinant vector vaccine—an experimental vaccine that uses attenuated virus or bacterium to introduce microbial DNA to cells of the body; the vector is the virus or bacterium that serves as the carrier

Reservoir host—the species that is the source of a disease; not all organisms in the species would be sources, but the species itself is capable of hosting the disease (see also, Carrier species)

Rotavirus—the number one reason for hospitalization admissions of children due to gastroenteritis in the United States

Smallpox—an infectious disease that was declared eradicated in 1979 through a worldwide vaccination effort; over 80 percent of infected children died from the disease

Subacute Sclerosing Panencephalitis (SSPE)—a rare and generally fatal measles complication

Subunit vaccine—a vaccine that does not contain the entire microbe, but instead, has just the antigens that do the best job of stimulating the immune system

Tetanus—a nerve disorder caused by the toxin of a common bacterium, it induces painful tightening of muscles all over the body.

Thimerosal—an ethylmercury-containing preservative in some vaccines

Toxoid—a deactivated toxin used as the basis for a vaccine against a toxin-based disease such as diphtheria or tetanus

Vaccination—a disease-prevention measure involving the use of antigenic material to stimulate a person's immune response, thereby triggering an acquired immunity to a particular disease

Variolation—a pre-vaccination technique used to prevent smallpox, it involved exposing an uninfected person to material from a smallpox blister

Endnotes

NOTES TO INTRODUCTION

1. "Public and Scientists' Views on Science and Society," Pew Research Center, January 29, 2015, 46.
2. Bernice L. Housman, Mecal Ghebremichael, Philip Hayek and Erin Mack, "Poisonous, Filthy, Loathsome, Damnable Stuff': The Rhetorical Ecology of Vaccination Concern," *Yale Journal of Biology and Medicine* 87(Dec 2014): 403–416, accessed April 16, 2015, http://www.ncbi.nlm.nih.gov/pmc/articles/PMC4257028/.
3. Eric Kodish, "The ethical negligence of parents who refuse to vaccinate their children," *The Washington Post*, June 26, 2014.

NOTES TO CHAPTER I

1. Matthew M. David (Poll Director), et al., "Parent view on medical research: safety of vaccines & medicines top priorities," C.S. Mott Children's Hospital National Poll on Children's Health, Vol 11 Issue 1, October 11, 2010, accessed May 5, 2015, http://mottnpch.org/reports-surveys/parent-views-medical-research-safety-vaccines-medicines-top-priorities.
2. Ibid.
3. Ibid.
4. "Does polio still exist? Is it curable?" World Health Organization website, last modified October 2014, http://www.who.int/features/qa/07/en/.

5. "What is Polio?" Centers for Disease Control and Prevention website, accessed May 6, 2015, http://www.cdc.gov/polio/about/.

6. "Measles in the Philippines," Centers for Disease Control and Prevention website, last modified March 25, 2015, http://wwwnc.cdc.gov/travel/notices/watch/measles-philippines.

7. Reem Sharhan, "Measles Around the World," *The Disease Daily*, July 5, 2013, accessed April 28, 2015, http://www.healthmap.org/site/disease daily/article/measles-around-world-7513.

8. Ibid.

9. Jason Wells, "Here's How Many Americans Have Contracted The Measles In The Disneyland Outbreak," Public Health Departments for Affected States as cited by *BuzzFeed News*, last modified February 26, 2015, http://www.buzzfeed.com/jasonwells/track-measles-outbreak-across-the-us#.igwxmmJBW.

10. Gareth Williams, "From Jenner to Wakefield: The long shadow of the anti-vaccination movement," delivered at Barnard's Inn Hall at Gresham College on September 28, 2011, accessed May 15, 2015, https://www.youtube.com/watch?v=YFauihFXKHk.

11. Jenny McCarthy interviewed by Kirin Chetry, *CNN*, November 26, 2012, accessed May 15, 2015, https://www.youtube.com/watch?v=-2bhQ3SYJhg.

12. "Sharing Personal Stories—Measles," Parents PACK, The Children's Hospital of Philadelphia website, accessed July 26, 2015, http://vec.chop.edu/service/parents-possessing-accessing-communicating-knowledge-about-vaccines/sharing-personal-stories/sharing-personal-story-measles.html.

13. Ibid.

14. Robert W. Sears, *The Vaccine Book* (New York: Little, Brown and Company, 2007), 238.

15. "The Deadliest Infectious Diseases," *Planet Deadly*, November 22, 2014, accessed August 26, 2015, http://www.planetdeadly.com/nature/deadliest-infectious-diseases.

16. "Western Hemisphere Wipes Out Its Third Virus," *All Things Considered*, National Public Radio, April 30, 2015, accessed August 26, 2015, http://www.npr.org/blogs/goatsandsoda/2015/04/30/403388700/western-hemisphere-wipes-out-its-third-virus.

17. The number of cases was not reported until the 1970 data collection effort, at which time there were 104,953 cases reported, so it is conservative to say that the number in 1960 exceeded 100,000.

18. The number of cases was not reported until the 1970 data collection effort, at which time there were 56,797 cases reported, so it is conservative to say that the number in 1960 exceeded 55,000.

19. The number of cases was not reported until the 1970 data collection effort, at which time there were 2,505 cases reported, with the trend in the next ten years on the rise, so it is conservative to say that the number in 1960 exceeded 2,500.

20. "Selected notifiable disease rates and number of new cases: United States, selected years 1950–2011," Health, United States, 2013, US Department of Health and Human Services, Centers for Disease Control and Prevention, National Center for Health Statistics, 2013, 145.

21. Lenny Bernstein and Rebecca Schatz, "Vaccine protester has change of heart," The Denver Post, April 16, 2015, 18A.

22. Ibid.

23. "Update: Adverse Events Following Smallpox Vaccination—United States, 2003, Centers for Disease Control and Prevention," CDC website, last modified April 3, 2003, http://www.cdc.gov/mmwr/preview/mmwrhtml/mm5213a4.htm.

24. Interview with Jim McCormick, founder and president of Research Institute for Risk Intelligence, April 13, 2015.

25. Benjamin J. Cowling, Vicky J. Fang, Hiroshi Nishirua, Kwok-Hung Chan, Sophia Ng, Dennis K. M. Ip, Susan S. Chiu, Gabriel M. Leung and J.S. Malik Peiris, "Increased risk of non-influenza respiratory virus infections associated with receipt of inactivated influenza vaccine," Clinical Infectious Diseases, Oxford University Press, March 15, 2012, accessed July 15, 2015, http://cid.oxfordjournals.org/content/early/2012/03/13/cid.cis307.full.pdf+html.

26. Ibid.

27. FDA website archives, http://www.casewatch.org/fdawarning/prod/2006/mercola2.shtml and http://www.fda.gov/ICECI/EnforcementActions/WarningLetters/2011/ucm250701.htm.

28. This is an annotated list, using language from the Mayo Clinic website to describe some conditions in layman's terms, of Joseph Mercola's list in "Vaccines and Neurological Damage," http://www.mercola.com/article/vaccines/neurological_damage.htm.

29. "Mesothelioma," Mayo Clinic website, accessed August 1, 2015, http://www.mayoclinic.org/diseases-conditions/mesothelioma/basics/risk-factors/con-20026157?_ga=1.92429277.173587238.1429229051.

30. James J. Sejvar, "Vaccines and Neurologic Disease," *Seminars in Neurology* 31(2011):338–355, accessed April 16, 2015, http://www.medscape.com/viewarticle/751103_2.

31. Ibid.

NOTES TO CHAPTER 2

1. "Hepatitis B Vaccine History," Hepatitis B Foundation website, last modified October 21, 2009, http://www.hepb.org/professionals/hepatitis_b_vaccine.htm.

2. Ibid., http://www.hepb.org/patients/general_information.htm.

3. Sears, *The Vaccine Book*, 49 and 237.

4. Ibid., 174.

5. World Health Organization website, http://apps.who.int/immunization_monitoring/globalsummary/timeseries/tsincidencediphtheria.html.

6. "What is Tetanus?" WebMD website, last modified March 11, 2015, http://www.webmd.com/a-to-z-guides/understanding-tetanus-basics.

7. Sears, *The Vaccine Book*, 173–174.

8. "What is Tetanus?" WebMD.

9. CDC and WebMD websites, http://www.cdc.gov/pertussis/pregnant/mom/get-vaccinated.html and http://www.webmd.com/parenting/baby/features/protect-baby-whooping-cough.

10. "Vaccine Information Statement – DTaP (Tetanus, Diphtheria, Pertussis) Vaccine: What you need to know," Department of Health and Human Services, Centers for Disease Control and Prevention, (5/17/2007), 42 U.S.C. § 300aa-26.

11. "Genetics Home Reference," National Institutes of Health, August 2012; http://ghr.nlm.nih.gov/condition/cystic-fibrosis.

12. Centers for Disease Control and Prevention, "Prevalence of Duchenne/Beckermuscular dystrophy among males aged 5-24 years—four states, 2007," MMWR Morbidity and Mortality Weekly Report, 58, 1119-1122 (2009), http://www.cdc.gov/mmwr/preview/mmwrhtml/mm5840a1.htm.

13. "Haemophilus Influenzae Type b (Hib) VIS," Vaccine Information Statements, Centers for Disease Control and Prevention, April 2, 2015, http://www.cdc.gov/vaccines/hcp/vis/vis-statements/hib.html.

14. Matthew P. Rubach, Jeffrey M. Bender, Susan Mottice, Kimberly Hanson, Hsin Yi Cindy Weng, Kent Korgenski, Judy A. Daly and Andrew T. Pavia, "Increasing Incidence of Invasive *Haemophilus influenza* Disease in Adults, Utah, USA," *Emerging Infectious Diseases*, Volume 17, Number

9 (September 2011), accessed July 5, 2015, http://wwwnc.cdc.gov/eid/article/17/9/10–1991_article.

15. Sears, *The Vaccine Book*, 224.

16. "Famous People who had and have Polio," *Disabled World*, accessed August 26, 2015, http://www.disabled-world.com/artman/publish/famous-polio.shtml.

17. "Does polio still exist? Is it curable?" World Health Organization website, accessed May 20, 2015, http://www.who.int/features/qa/07/en/.

18. RotaTeq (Rotavirus Vaccine) Questions and Answers, Food and Drug Administration website, accessed August 2, 2015, http://www.fda.gov/BiologicsBloodVaccines/Vaccines/QuestionsaboutVaccines/ucm100242.htm.

19. L. Simonsen, C. Viboud, A. Elixhauser, R.J. Taylora and A.Z. Kapikian, "More on RotaShield and Intussesception: The Role of Age at the Time of Vaccination," *The Journal of Infectious Diseases*, Volume 192, Issue Supplement1, S36-S43, accessed April 16, 2015, http://jid.oxfordjournals.org/content/192/Supplement_1/S36.full.

20. "Important Safety Information," last modified November 2012, www.menactra.com.

21. Mayo Clinic Stagg, "Autism spectrum disorder," Mayo Clinic website, accessed June 24, 2015, http://www.mayoclinic.org/diseases-conditions/autism-spectrum-disorder/basics/symptoms/con-20021148.

22. "Patient Information RotaTeq," Merck Sharp & Dohme Corp, last modified June 2013, http://www.merck.com/product/usa/pi_circulars/r/rotateq/rotateq_ppi.pdf.

23. Sears, *The Vaccine Book*, 239.

24. Ibid.

25. Stephanie Cave, "Recommended Vaccine Schedule," Children'sHealth Choices.org, accessed July 13, 2015, http://childrenshealthchoices.org/cave.html.

26. Catherine Saint Louis, "Most Doctors Give In to Requests by Parents to Alter Vaccine Schedules," *The New York Times*, March 2, 2015, accessed August 11, 2015, http://www.nytimes.com/2015/03/02/science/most-doctors-give-in-to-requests-by-parents-to-alter-vaccine-schedules.html?_r=0.

27. "Questions about Altering the Recommended Vaccine Schedule," The Children's Hospital of Philadelphia Parents PACK, accessed April 14, 2015, http://vec.chop.edu/service/parents-possessing-accessing-commun

icating-knowledge-about-vaccines/vaccines-schedule/questions-about
-altering-the-schedule.html#alter-immunization-schedule.

28. PubMed search results for "Intussusception children RotaTeq," August 26, 2015, http://www.ncbi.nlm.nih.gov/pubmed/?term=intussu sception+children+RotaTeq.

29. W.K. Yih, T. A. Lieu, M. Kulldorff, D. Martin, C. N. McMahill-Walraven, R. Platt, N. Selvam, M. Selvan, G. M. Lee and M. Nguyen, "Intussusception risk after rotavirus vaccination in U.S. infants," *New England Journal of Medicine* 370 (February 6, 2014): 503–12, access date April 20, 2015, doi: 10.1056/NWJMoa 1303164, http://www.ncbi.nlm.nih.gov/pubmed/ 24422676.

30. "Vaccine Misconception of the day—Aluminum in vaccines," *Vaccine Central*, November 1, 2010, accessed March 24, 2015, https://vaccine-central.wordpress.com/2010/11/01/vaccine-misconception-of-the -day-aluminum-in-vaccines/.

31. "Aluminum in Vaccines: What you should know," The Children's Hospital of Philadelphia, *Q&A* Volume 5, Winter 2014, accessed April 2, 2015, http://vec.chop.edu/export/download/pdfs/articles/vaccine-education -center/aluminum.pdf.

NOTES TO CHAPTER 3

1. "The Development of the Immunization Schedule," The History of Vaccines website, an educational resource by The College of Physicians of Philadelphia, accessed May 13, 2015, http://www.historyofvaccines.org/ content/articles/development-immunization-schedule.

2. R. Austrian, "A brief history of pneumococcal vaccines," *Drugs & Aging*, 15 Suppl 1 (1999):1–10, accessed May 16, 2015, http://www.ncbi.nlm .nih.gov/pubmed/10690790.

3. "Nasal Spray Flu Vaccine in Children 2 through 8 Years Old," Centers for Disease Control and Prevention website, accessed July 18, 2015, http:// www.cdc.gov/flu/about/qa/nasalspray-children.htm.

4. Ibid.

5. J.D. Grabenstein, "Vaccine Excipient & Media Summary," *ImmunoFacts: Vaccines and Immunologic Drugs—2013* (38th revision), Wolters Kluwer Health.

6. "Nasal Spray Fly Vaccine," CDC.

7. "A Parent's Story of Vaccine Reaction," *Harpocrates Speaks*, August 5, 2011, accessed July 18, 2015, http://www.harpocratesspeaks.com/2011/08/parents-story-of-vaccine-reaction.html.

8. "Frequently Asked Questions on Syncope After Vaccination," Centers for Disease Control and Prevention website, accessed July 21, 2015, http://www.cdc.gov/vaccinesafety/Concerns/syncope_faqs.html.

9. Harald zur Hausen, "Harald zur Hausen—Biographical," Nobelprize.org, accessed July 24, 2015, http://www.nobelprize.org/nobel_prizes/medicine/laureates/2008/hausen-bio.html.

10. "AIDS pioneers and HPV cancer researcher win Nobel Prize for medicine or physiology," The Rockefeller University website, October 7, 2008, accessed July 29, 2015, http://librarynews.rockefeller.edu/?p=458.

11. "Human Papillomavirus," *The Pink Book*: Course Textbook—12th Edition Second Printing (May 2012), Centers for Disease Control and Prevention, 2, accessed July 25, 2015, http://www.cdc.gov/vaccines/pubs/pinkbook/hpv.html.

12. 2015 Immunization Schedules, American Academy of Pediatrics, accessed July 26, 2015, http://www2.aap.org/immunization/izschedule.html.

13. Ibid.

14. Catch-Up Immunization Scheduler, last modified March 3, 2014, https://www.vacscheduler.org/scheduler.html?v=patient.

15. "A Parent's Story," *Harpocrates Speaks*.

16. Paul H. Patterson, *Infectious Behavior: Brain-Immune Connections in Autism, Schizophrenia, and Depression*, (Cambridge: The MIT Press, 2011), 109.

17. This is the 2008 Census Bureau figure.

18. Richard Feldman, "No medical research proves vaccine, autism link," *The Indianapolis Star*, April 14, 2014, accessed June 29, 2015, http://www.indystar.com/story/opinion/2014/04/14/medical-research-proves-vaccine-autism-link/7707323/.

19. Fangjun Zhou, Ph.D., Jeanne Santoli, M.D., M.P.H., Mark L. Messonnier, Ph.D., Hussain R. Yusuf, M.B.B.S., M.P.H., Abigail Shefer, M.D., Susan Y. Chu, Ph.D., M.S.P.H., Lance Rodewald, M.D. and Rafael Harpaz, M.D., M.P.H., "Econoomic Evaluation of the 7-Vaccine Routine Childhood Immunization Schedule in the United States, 2001," *Archives of Pediatrics and Adolescent Medicine* (Reprinted) Vol 159, Dec 2005, accessed May 24, 2015, http://www.317coalition.org/documents/moreresources16.pdf.

NOTES TO CHAPTER 4

1. Sinead M. Langan, Liam Smeeth, David J. Margolis and Sara L. Thomas, "Herpes Zoster Vaccine Effectiveness against Incident Herpes Zoster and Post-herpetic Neuralgia in an Older US Population: A Cohort Study," *PLOS Medicine*, April 9, 2013, accessed July 14, 2015, doi: 10,1371/journal.pmed.1001420, http://journals.plos.org/plosmedicine/article?id =10.1371/journal.pmed.1001420.

2. Walter W. Williams, M.D., Peng-Jun Lu, M.D., Ph.D., Alissa O'Halloran, M.S.P.H., Carolyn B. Bridges, M.D.,Tamara Pilishvili, M.P.H., Craig M. Hales, M.D. and Lauri E. Markowitz, M.D., "Noninfluenza Vaccination Coverage Among Adults—United States, 2012," Morbidity and Mortality Weekly Report, Centers for Disease Control and Prevention website, February 7, 2014, accessed July 24, 2015, http://www.cdc.gov/mmwr/preview/mmwrhtml/mm6305a4.htm.

3. Joe Neel, "How Many People Die From Flu Each Year? Depends on How You Slice The Data," *National Public Radio*, August 26, 2010, accessed August 10, 2015, http://www.npr.org/blogs/health/2010/08/26/129456 941/annual-flu-death-average-fluctuates-depending-on-how-you -slice-it.

4. "Flu Vaccination Coverage, United States, 2012–2013 Influenza Season," Centers for Disease Control and Protection website, accessed August 20, 2015, http://www.cdc.gov/flu/fluvaxview/coverage-1213 estimates.htm#age-group.

5. Langan, et al., "Herpes Zoster Vaccine Effectiveness."

6. Eula Biss as interviewed by Audie Cornish, "Vaccine Controversies Area As Social As They Are Medical," *National Public Radio*, September 30, 2014, accessed July 25, 2015, http://www.npr.org/blogs/health/2014/09/30/351242264/vaccine-controversies-are-as -social-as-they-are-medical.

7. Sears, *The Vaccine Book*, 247.

8. Keli Rabon, Jason Foster and Phil Tenser, "How many students are unvaccinated in your child's school? Check data from local school districts," *ABC 7 News Denver* and *The Denver Post*, February 11, 2015, accessed April 17, 2015, http://www.thedenverchannel.com/lifestyle/education/how-many-students-are-unvaccinated-in-your-childs-school -check-data-from-local-school-districts.

9. Arthur Allen, "Bucking the Herd," *The Atlantic*, September 2002, accessed May 4, 2015, http://www.theatlantic.com/magazine/archive/2002/09/bucking-the-herd/302556/.

10. "Seasonal Influenza Vaccine Effectiveness, 2005–2015," Centers for Disease Control and Prevention website, accessed May 17, 2015, http://www.cdc.gov/flu/professionals/vaccination/effectiveness-studies .htm.

11. Benjamin J. Cowling, et al., "Increased risk of non-influenza respiratory virus infections."

12. "Pneumococcal Disease," *The History of Vaccines*, last modified December 31, 2014, http://www.historyofvaccines.org/content/articles/pneumococcal-disease-0.

NOTES TO CHAPTER 5

1. Carrie Cariello, "I Know What Causes Autism," January 19, 2015, accessed April 20, 2015, http://carriecariello.com/2015/01/19/i-know-what-causes-autism/.

2. Kristian Sjogren, "Study links autism with circumcision," *ScienceNordic*, January 15, 2015, accessed April 21, 2015, http://sciencenordic.com/study-links-autism-circumcision.

3. Morten Frisch and Jacob Simonsen, "Ritual circumcision and risk of autism spectrum disorder in 0- to 9-year-old boys: national cohort study in Denmark," *Journal of The Royal Society of Medicine*, J R Soc Med, January 8, 2015, accessed April 21, 2015, http://jrs.sagepub.com/content/early/2015/01/07/0141076814565942.full.

4. "Pain and Your Infant: Medical Procedures, Circumcision and Teething," University of Michigan Health System, accessed May 1, 2015, http://www.med.umich.edu/yourchild/topics/paininf.htm.

5. Cariello, "I Know What Causes Autism."

6. Seth Mnookin, author of *The Panic Virus: A True Story of Medicine, Science and Fear*, on a panel "Vaccines and Autism: A Story of Medicine, Science and Fear," *The Diane Rehm Show*, National Public Radio, February 2, 2011, accessed April 22, 2015, http://thedianerehmshow.org/shows/2011–02–02/vaccines-and-autism-story-medicine -science-and-fear.

7. Alison Tepper Singer, Founder and President of the Autism Science Foundation, on a panel "Vaccines and Autism: A Story of Medicine, Science and Fear," *The Diane Rehm Show*, National Public Radio, February 2, 2011;, accessed April 22, 2015, http://thedianerehmshow.org/shows/2011–02–02/vaccines-and-autism-story-medicine -science-and-fear.

8. Roberta DeBiasi, pediatric infectious diseases physician at Children's National Medical Center, on a panel "Vaccines and Autism: A Story of Medicine, Science and Fear," *The Diane Rehm Show, National Public Radio*, February 2, 2011, April 22, 2015, http://thedianerehm show.org/shows/2011–02–02/vaccines-and-autism-story-medicine -science-and-fear.

9. "History of Autism," WebMD website, accessed April 24, 2015, http:// www.webmd.com/brain/autism/history-of-autism.

10. Paul H. Patterson, *Infectious Behavior: Brain-Immune Connections in Autism, Schizophrenia, and Depression* (Cambridge: MIT Press, 2011), 108.

11. Ibid.

12. Pat Levitt, Ph.D., in an email to Maryann Karinch, April 28, 2015

13. Jeffrey S. Gerber and Paul A. Offit, "Vaccines and Autism: A Tale of Shifting Hypotheses," *Clinical Infectious Diseases*, 48–456–61 (2009), accessed April 25, 2015, doi: 10.1086/596475.

14. Jenny McCarthy, "In the Vaccine-Autism Debate, What Can Parents Believe?," *The Huffington Post*, January 10, 2011, updated May 25, 2011, accessed April 25, 2015, http://www.huffingtonpost.com/ jenny-mccarthy/vaccine-autism-debate_b_806857.html.

15. Joseph Mercola, "Is Alarming Rise in Autism Linked to 1988 Event?" Mercola.com, November 15, 2011, accessed April 26, 2015, http://articles.mercola.com/sites/articles/archive/2011/11/15/ vaccines-behind-autism-epidemic.aspx.

16. Gerber and Offit, "Vaccines and Autism," 7.

17. "About," International Medical Council on Vaccination website, accessed July 19, 2015, www.vaccinationcouncil.org/about.

18. "Quick Compare," International Medical Council on Vaccination web-site, accessed July 19, 2015, http://www.vaccinationcouncil.org/quick -compare-2/.

19. "The PA Amish Lifestyle," *Discover Lancaster*, accessed July 20, 2015, http://www.discoverlancaster.com/towns-and-heritage/amish-country/ amish-lifestyle.asp.

20. H. Honda, Y. Shimizu and M. Rutter, "No effect of MMR withdrawal on the incidence of autism: a total population study," *Journal of Child Psychology and Psychiatry* 46(June 2005):572–9, accessed July 23, 2015, http://www.ncbi.nlm.nih.gov/pubmed/15877763.

21. K. Angkustsiri, D. D. Li and R. Hansen, "No Differences in Early Immunization Rates among Children with Typical Development and

Autism Spectrum Disorders," International Society for Autism Research, May 2, 2013, accessed May 5, 2015, https://imfar.confex.com/imfar/2013/webprogram/Paper12796.html.

22. Autism Web Forum, accessed May 5, 2015, http://www.autismweb.com/forum/viewtopic.php?f=6&t=30749.

23. Statement of William W. Thompson, Ph.D., Regarding the 2004 Article Examining the Possibility of a Relationship between MMR Vaccine and Autism, issued by Morgan Verkamp, LLC, Cincinnati, Ohio, accessed May 13, 2015, http://www.morganverkamp.com/.

24. Letter from William W. Thompson, Ph.D. to former CDC director Dr. Julie Gerberding, February 2, 2004.

25. Sharyl Attkisson, "Family to Receive $1.5M+ in First-Ever Vaccine-Autism Court Award," *CBS News*, September 10, 2010, accessed July 1, 2015, http://www.cbsnews.com/news/family-to-receive-15m-plus-in-first-ever-vaccine-autism-court-award/.

26. Julie Gerberding as quoted in "Vaccine case draws new attention to autism debate," *CNN*, March 7, 2008, accessed July 1, 2015, http://www.cnn.com/2008/HEALTH/conditions/03/06/vaccines.autism/index.html.

27. O.M. Dekkers, M. Egger, D.G. Altman and J.P. Vandenbroucke, "Distinguishing case series from cohort studies," *Annals of Internal Medicine* 15(January 3, 2012): 37–40, accessed July 2, 2015, doi: 10.7326/0003–4819–156–1–201201030–00006, http://www.ncbi.nlm.nih.gov/pubmed/22213493.

28. A. Jain, J. Marshall, A. Buikema, T. Bancroft, J.P. Kelly and C.J. Newschaffer, "Autism occurrence by MMR vaccine status among US children with older siblings with and without autism," *JAMA* 313 (April 21, 2015):1534–40, accessed July 5, 2015, doi: 10.1001/jama.2015.3077, http://www.ncbi.nlm.nih.gov/pubmed/25898051.

29. Gerber and Offit,"Vaccines and Autism," 2.

30. "Cohort profile: The Norwegian Mother and Child Cohort Study (MoBa)," *International Journal of Epidemiology* Volume 35, Issue 5, 1146-1150, http://ije.oxfordjournals.org/content/35/5/1146.full.

NOTES TO CHAPTER 6

1. "Phenol," Merriam-Webster Dictionary Online, accessed August 26, 2015, http://www.merriam-webster.com/dictionary/phenol.

2. "Glycine," WebMD website, accessed August 26, 2015, http://www
   .webmd.com/vitamins-supplements/ingredientmono-1072-glycine
   .aspx?activeingredientid=1072&activeingredientname=glycine.

3. "Vaccine Excipient & Media Summary" from *ImmunoFacts: Vaccines and Immunologic Drugs—2013* (38th revision), St. Louis, MO, Wolters Kluwer Health, compiled by J.D. Grabenstein.

4. Ibid.

5. Gardiner Harris, "Government Says 2 Common Materials Pose Risk of Cancer," *The New York Times*, June 10, 2011.

6. "Vaccines and Formaldehyde," Vaccine Education Center website, The Children's Hospital of Philadelphia, accessed June 15, 2015, http://vec.chop.edu/service/vaccine-education-center/vaccine-safety/vaccine-ingredients/formaldehyde.html.

7. Deanna Blanchard, "The Vaccination Debate—Part 1: Dangerous Ingredients in Your Child's Vacciness That Your Doctor Probably WON'T Tell You About," SelfGrowth.com, accessed July 20, 2015, http://www.selfgrowth.com/articles/the_vaccination_debate_%E2%80%93_part_1_dangerous_ingredients_in_your_childs_vaccines_that_your_doc.

8. "Hydrogen," The Free Dictionary website, accessed August 3, 2015, http://www.thefreedictionary.com/hydrogen.

9. Example: Robert L. Coffman, Alan Sher and Robert A. Seder, "Vaccine Adjuvants: Putting Innate Immunity to Work", *Immunity*, Volume 33, Issue 4, 492–503, October 29, 2010, accessed August 4, 2015, http://www.nytimes.com/2011/06/11/health/11cancer.html?_r=0.

10. Sears, *The Vaccine Book*, 204.

11. Ibid., 7.

12. Lucija Tomljenovic and Christopher Shaw, "Aluminum Vaccine Adjuvants: Are They Safe?" *Current Medicinal Chemistry*, Volume 18, Number 17, June 2011, 2630–2637(8).

13. "Review of a published report of cerebral vasculitis after vaccination with the Human Papillomavirus (HPV) Vaccine," CDC-CISA Working Group Technical Report, Centers for Disease and Prevention website, November 9, 2012, accessed August 5, 2015, http://www.cdc.gov/vaccinesafety/Activities/cisa/technical_report.html.

14. Daniel Krewski, Robert A. Yokel, Evert Nieboer, David Borchelt, Joshua Cohen, Jean Harry, Sam Kacew, Joan Lindsay, Amal M. Mahfouz and Virginie Rondeau, "Human Health Risk Assessment For Aluminium, Aluminium Oxide, And Aluminium Hydroxide," *Journal of Toxicology and Environmental Health B Crit Rev.* 10 Suppl 1 (2007): 1–269, accessed

August 5, 2015, doi: 10.1080/10937400701597766, http://www.ncbi
.nlm.nih.gov/pmc/articles/PMC2782734/.

15. "Study Reports Aluminum in Vaccines Poses Extremely Low Risk to
Infants," U.S. Food and Drug Administration website, accessed July 25,
2015, http://www.fda.gov/BiologicsB.../ScienceResearch/ucm284520
.htm.

16. Ibid.

17. Richard Van Noorden, "Record number of journals banned for boosting
impact factor with self-citations," *Nature News*, June 29, 2012, accessed
June 29, 2015, http://blogs.nature.com/news/2012/06/record-number-
of-journals-banned-for-boosting-impact-factor-with-self-citations.html.

18. "Thimerosal in Vaccines," U.S. Food and Drug Administration website,
accessed June 29, 2015, http://www.fda.gov/BiologicsBloodVaccines/
SafetyAvailability/VaccineSafety/UCM096228.

19. "Frequently Asked Questions about Thimerosal," Centers for Disease
Control and Prevention website, accessed July 15, 2015, http://www.cdc
.gov/vaccinesafety/Concerns/thimerosal/thimerosal_faqs.html#b.

20. L.K. Ball, R. Ball and R.D. Pratt, "An assessment of thimerosal use in
childhood vaccines," *Pediatrics* 107(May 2001):1147–54.

21. Ibid.

22. Robert F. Kennedy, Jr. and Mark Hyman, "Thimerosal: Let the Science
Speak," White Paper (2014), accessed May 15, 2015, http://www
.autisminvestigated.com/wp-content/uploads/2014/07/Thimerosal
_Kennedy.doc.

23. Gardiner Harris and Anahad O'Connor, "On Autism's Cause, It's Parents
vs. Research," *The New York Times*, June 26, 2005, accessed May 28, 2015,
http://www.nytimes.com/2005/06/25/science/25autism.html?page
wanted=print&_r=0.

24. K.M. Madsen, M.B. Lauritsen, C.B. Pedersen, P. Thorsen, A.M. Plesner,
P.H. Andersen and P.B. Mortensen, "Thimerosal and the occurrence of
autism: negative ecological evidence from Danish population-based
data," *Pediatrics*, 112 (September 2003):604–6.

25. Thomas H. Maugh II and Andrew Zajac, "'Vaccines court' rejects
mercury-autism link in 3 test cases," *Los Angeles Times*, March 13, 2010.

26. Kennedy, Jr. and Hyman, "Thimerosal: Let the Science Speak."

NOTES TO CHAPTER 7

1. Dirk Johnson, "Trials for Parents who Chose Faith Over Medicine," *The New York Times*, January 20, 2009, accessed June 1, 2015, http://www .nytimes.com/2009/01/21/us/21faith.html?_r=0.

2. Carey Goldberg, "Research: Could Birth-Canal Bacteria Help C-Section Babies?" *WBUR, National Public Radio*, June 25, 2014, accessed June 1, 2015, http://commonhealth.wbur.org/2014/06/birth-canal -bacteria-c-section.

3. Dr. Maria Gloria Dominguez-Bello interviewed by Carey Goldberg for *WBUR, National Public Radio*, June 25, 2014.

4. L.A. Hanson, "Breastfeeding provides passive and likely long-lasting active immunity," *Annals of Allergy, Asthma, and Immunology* 81(December 1998):523–33, accessed July 3, 2015, http://www.ncbi.nlm.nih.gov/ pubmed/9892025.

5. Recorded interview with Lacey Grabel, March 22, 2015.

6. Rabon, Foster and Tenser, "How many students are unvaccinated in your child's school?"

7. X. Li, et al., "Immunogenetic influences on acquisition of HIV-1 infection: consensus findings from two African cohorts point to an enhancer element in *IL19* (1q32.2)," *Genes & Immunity* 16 (2015): 213–220, accessed July 7, 2015, doi:10.1038/gene.2014.84, http://www.nature.com/gene/ journal/v16/n3/full/gene201484a.html.

8. N. A. Davis, J. E. Crowe Jr., N. M. Pajewski and B. A. McKinney, "Surfing a genetic association interaction network to identify modulators of antibody response to smallpox vaccine," *Genes & Immunity* 11 (2010): 630– 636, accessed July 17, 2015, doi:10.1038/gene.2010.37, http://www .nature.com/gene/journal/v11/n8/abs/gene201037a.html.

9. "Vaccine Injury Compensation: Most Claims Took Multiple Years and Many Were Settled through Negotiation," Report of the U.S. Government Accountability Office, GAO-15-142, published: Nov 21, 2014, accessed July 18, 2015, http://www.gao.gov/products/GAO-15-142.

10. Yasuko Fukuda as quoted by Lydia O'Connor, "Do Not Bring Your Kids To 'Measles Parties,' Doctors Warn," *Huffington Post*, February 11, 2015, accessed August 5, 2015, http://www.huffingtonpost.com/2015/02/11/ measles-parties-warning_n_6658232.html.

11. Melinda Wenner Moyer, "What to Do if You Get Invited to a Chickenpox Party (Don't go)," Slate.com, November 15, 2013, accessed June 25, 2015, http://www.slate.com/articles/double_x/the_kids/2013/11/chicken pox_vaccine_is_it_really_necessary.html.

12. Shane Ellison, "Herd Immunity: Three Reasons Why I Don't Vaccinate My Children...And Why Vaccine Supporters Shouldn't Care That I Use Vaccine Exemption Forms," *The People's Chemist*, accessed July 19, 2015, http://thepeopleschemist.com/reasons-dont-vaccinate-children -vaccine-supporters-shouldnt-give/.

NOTE TO CHAPTER 8

1. Diderik Finne, M.S., Lac, C.C.H, "Homeoprophylaxis: Better than Vaccination?" accessed July 25, 2015, http://home.mindspring.com/ ~diderikfinne/homeoprophylaxis.pdf.

2. John Stossel, "Stossel: Homeopathic Remedies," *ABC News*, January 30, 2012, accessed July 25, 2015, http://abcnews.go.com/2020/GiveMe ABreak/story?id=124309&page=1.

3. James Randi and Dana Ullman were pitted against each other in an "experiment" done by ABC's *20/20*, however, this was a contrived event and proved nothing about either homeopathy or the legitimacy of skepticism.

4. Andrew Weil, "Homeopathic Medicine," Dr.Weil.com, accessed July 26, 2015, http://www.drweil.com/drw/u/ART00470/Homeopathic-Medicine .html.

5. Homeopathy Plus website, accessed August 1, 2015, http://homeopathy plus.com.au/.

6. "FDA Ponders Putting Homeopathy to a Tougher Test," *National Public Radio*, April 20, 2015, accessed July 30, 2015, http://www.npr.org/tem plates/transcript/transcript.php?storyId=398806514.

7. Peter Fisher, "Does Homeopathy Work?" a debate with Dr. Ben Goldacre at the Natural History Museum in London, March 23, 2012, accessed July 30, 2015, https://www.youtube.com/watch?v=DKEtHtl97D0.

8. James Randi, "Homeopathy, quackery and fraud," TED2007, February 2007, Monterey, California, accessed August 1, 2015, http://www.ted .com/talks/james_randi#t-754304.

9. The 10:23 Challenge involved protestors from 70 cities (30 countries) who gathered in their respective locations to take "overdoses" of homeopathic remedies in an effort to disprove their merits. See: http://www.1023.org. uk/the-1023-challenge.php. It was an event of the Merseyside Skeptics Society, a group devoted to so-called scientific skepticism (http://www. merseysideskeptics.org.uk/).

10. "Uses and Warnings," Hyland's Calms Forté Product Information, October 2008, accessed July 25, 2015, http://www.calmsforte.com/home/2008/10/uses-warnings/.

11. "Tutorial 1—The Law of Similars," Homeopathy Plus website, accessed August 1, 2015, http://homeopathyplus.com.au/tutorial-1-the-law-of-similars/.

12. Dana Ullman, "The Cutting Edge of Science, Homeopathy and Nanomedicine—Part I (of V)," presentation to The Commonweath Club, San Francisco, September 17, 2014, accessed August 3, 2015, https://www.youtube.com/watch?v=ZVKuqrHbuwk.

13. Ibid., Part III.

14. *National Geographic* website, accessed May 1, 2015, http://animals.nationalgeographic.com/animals/fish/great-white-shark/.

15. Thomas Kruzel, N.D., *Natural Medicine Pediatric Home* (Self-Published 2012), 98.

16. Cilla Whatcott, "How Homeoprophylaxis Educates the Immune System," The Solution—Homeoprophylaxis: The Vaccine Alternative, February 23, 2014, accessed July 24, 2015, http://hpsolution.org/2014/02/23/how-homeoprophylaxis-educates-the-immune-system-2/.

17. Finne, et al., "Homeoprophylaxis: Better than Vaccination?"

18. H.U. Albonico, H.U. Bräker and J. Hüsler, "Febrile infectious childhood diseases in the history of cancer patients and matched controls," *Medical Hypotheses*, 51(October 1998): 315–20, accessed July 30, 2015, http://www.ncbi.nlm.nih.gov/pubmed/9824838.

19. Mehar S. Manku, Medical Hypothesis Forum, *Elsevier*, accessed August 4, 2015, http://www.journals.elsevier.com/medical-hypotheses/.

20. The post to which it refers now results in a 404 error, because the content was removed.

21. "Shingles Goes Epidemic: Chicken Pox Vax to Blame," *The Liberty Beacon*, March 6, 2013, accessed August 11, 2015, http://www.thelibertybeacon.com/2013/03/06/shingles-goes-epidemic-chicken-pox-vax-to-blame/.

22. Dana Ullman, "Comments on the Vaccine Issue," Frequency Research Foundation, January 27, 2013, accessed July 30, 2015, http://blog.frequencyfoundation.com/2013/01/dana-ullman-on-vaccines-with-references.html.

23. "Measles and the Vaccine (Shot) to Prevent It," Centers for Disease Control and Prevention website, accessed April 20, 2015, http://www.cdc.gov/vaccines/vpd-vac/measles/fs-parents.html.

NOTES TO CHAPTER 9

1. "Vaccination Coverage Among Children in Kindergarten—United States, 2013–14 School Year," Centers for Disease Control and Prevention, *MMWR* 63 (October 17, 2014): 913–920.

2. Alex B. Berezow, "Are Liberals or Conservatives More Anti-Vaccine?" *Real Clear Science*, October 20, 2014, accessed August 3, 2015, http://www.real clearscience.com/journal_club/2014/10/20/are_liberals_or_conservatives _more_anti-vaccine_108905.html.

3. Tracy A. Lieu, G. Thomas Ray, Nicola P. Klein, Cindy Chung and Martin Kuldorff, "Geographic Clusters in Underimmunization and Vaccine Refusal," *Pediatrics*, January 19, 2015, accessed August 5, 2015, doi: 10.1542/peds.2014–2715.

4. Ibid.

5. "Personal Beliefs Exemption to Required Immunizations," California Department of Public Health, accessed August 4, 2015, http://eziz.org/ assets/docs/CDPH-8262.pdf.

6. Greg Miller, "Why the 'Prius Driving, Composting' Set Fears Vaccines", *Science*, January 2011, accessed August 10, 2015, http://news.science mag/2011/01/why-prius-driving-composting-set-fears-vaccines.

7. Ibid.

8. Ibid.

9. Jennifer A. Reich, "Neoliberal Mothering and Vaccine Refusal," *Gender & Society*, September 2, 2014, accessed August 12, 2015, https:// gendersociety.wordpress.com/2014/09/02/neoliberal-mothering -and-vaccine-refusal/.

10. Rachel Hills, "The Best Way to Combat Anti-Vaxxers Is to Understand Them," *New Republic*, January 5, 2015, accessed August 12, 2015, http://www.newrepublic.com/article/120695/study-anti-vaccination- supporters-practice-neoliberal-mothering.

11. Jennifer A. Reich, "Neoliberal Mothering and Vaccine Refusal."

12. Stephan Lewandowsky, Gilles E. Gignac and Klaus Oberauer, "The Role of Conspiracist Ideation and Worldviews in Predicting Rejection of Science," *PLOS ONE*, October 2, 2013, accessed August 13, 2015, doi: 10.1371/ journal.pone.0075637, http://journals.plos.org/plosone/article?id= 10.1371/journal.pone.0075637.

13. "Human Cell Strains in Vaccine Development," The History of Vaccines, College of Physicians of Philadelphia, accessed August 13, 2015, http:// www.historyofvaccines.org/content/articles/human-cell-strains -vaccine-development.

14. "FAQ on the Use of Vaccines," National Catholic Bioethics Center, accessed August 14, 2015, http://www.ncbcenter.org/page.aspx?pid =1284#assocAbort.

15. "KNOW...Religious Conviction," Vaccine Awareness of Northern Florida, accessed August 15, 2015, http://www.know-vaccines.org/ ?page_id=247.

16. Dr. James Todd, as quoted by Electra Draper, "Colorado vaccination law lacks enforcement, and no change is in works," *The Denver Post*, March 18, 2015, accessed August 15, 2015, http://www.denverpost .com/news/ci_27738009/colorado-vaccination-law-lacks-enforcement -and-no-change.

17. "Debate Over Vaccine Requirements Forges Strange Alliance," *The Associated Press*, February 6, 2015, accessed August 16, 2015, http:// www.nytimes.com/aponline/2015/02/06/us/ap-us-measles-vaccines -states.html?_r=0.

18. Lewandowsky, et al., "The Role of Conspiracist Ideation."

19. Gregory Hartley and Maryann Karinch, *The Most Dangerous Business Book You'll Ever Read* (Hoboken: John Wiley & Sons, 2011), 14.

20. Stephanie Saul and Andrew Pollack, "Furor on Rush to Require Cervical Cancer Vaccine," *The New York Times*, February 17, 2007, accessed August 18, 2015, http://www.nytimes.com/2007/02/17/health/17vaccine. html?pagewanted=all.

21. Amy Mitchell, Jeffrey Gottfried, Jocelyn Kiley and Katerina Eva Matsa, "Political Polarization & Media Habits," Pew Research Center Journalism and Media, accessed August 18, 2015, http://www.journalism .org/2014/10/21/political-polarization-media-habits/.

22. "A Necessary Vaccine," *The New York Times*, February 26, 2007, accessed August 18, 2015, http://www.nytimes.com/2007/02/26/opinion/ 26mon1.html.

23. Jonathan D. Rockoff, "Making Gardasil Vaccination Mandatory Would be Unwise, Academics Say," *Wall Street Journal Health Blog*, November 11, 2008, accessed August 17, 2015, http://blogs.wsj.com /health/2008/11/11/making-gardasil-vaccination-mandatory-would -be-unwise-academics-say/.

24. Ibid., quote from Gail Javitt of Johns Hopkins's Berman Institute of Bioethics.

25. Matthew Harper, "The Gardasil Problem: How the U.S. Lost Faith in a Promising Vaccine," *Forbes*, April 4, 2012, accessed August 20, 2015,

http://www.forbes.com/sites/matthewherper/2012/04/04/americas
-gardasil-problem-how-politics-poisons-public-health/.

26. Dan M. Kahan, Donald Braman, Geoffrey L. Cohen, John Gastil and
Paul Slovic, "Who Fears the HPV Vaccine, Who Doesn't, and Why? An
Experimental Study of the Mechanisms of Cultural Cognition," *Law &
Human Behavior* 34 (2010): 501–16, accessed August 21, 2015, http://
ssrn.com/abstract=1160654.

27. Ibid., 7.

28. Ibid., 11–12.

29. Mary Douglas, "A History of Grid and Group Cultural Theory" (lecture),
accessed May 10, 2015, http://projects.chass.utoronto.ca/semiotics/
cyber/douglas1.pdf.

30. Kahan, Braman, Cohen, Gastil and Slovic, "Who Fears the HPV Vaccine,
Who Doesn't, and Why?," 20.

31. Ibid., 25.

NOTES TO CHAPTER 10

1. "Medicines in Development for Vaccines," PhRMA, April 20, 2012,
accessed August 22, 2015, http://www.phrma.org/media/releases/
nearly-300-vaccines-development-prevention-treatment-disease.

2. Centers for Disease Control and Prevention website, accessed May 20,
2015, http://www.cdc.gov/vaccines/resdev/test-approve.htm.

3. Stanley Plotkin in a video on "The Future of Immunization," *The History
of Vaccines*, accessed August 23, 2015, http://www.historyofvaccines.
org/content/articles/future-immunization.

4. "Types of Vaccines," National Institute of Allergy and Infectious Diseases,
accessed August 23, 2015, http://www.niaid.nih.gov/topics/vaccines/
understanding/pages/typesvaccines.aspx.

5. Kishwar Hayat Khan, "DNA vaccines: roles against disease," Gemr 3(March
2013): 26–25, accessed August 24, 2015, doi: 10.11599/germs.2013:
1034, http://www.ncbi.nlm.nih.gov/pmc/articles/PMC3882840/.

6. Ibid., the complete lists of advantages and disadvantages are contained
in Tables 1 and 2 in the article.

7. WHO Media Centre Malaria, Fact sheet No.94., 2012, accessed August 25,
2015, http://www.who.int/mediacentre/factsheets/fs094/en/.

8. Ibid.

9. Ibid.

10. Plotkin, "The Future of Immunization."

11. World Health Organization website, accessed May 25, 2015, http://www. who.int/mediacentre/factsheets/fs380/en/.

12. Vincent Touhy, as quoted in a Cleveland Clinic video after Dr. Touhy was awarded the 2010 Sones Innovation Award, accessed August 26, 2015, http://giving.ccf.org/site/PageServer?pagename=vaccine.

13. Vincent Touhy, et al., "An autoimmune-mediated strategy for prophylactic breast cancer vaccination," *Nature Medicine* 16 (April 27, 2010): 799–803, accessed August 26, 2015, doi: 10.1038/nm.2161, http://www .nature.com/nm/journal/v16/n7/full/nm.2161.html.

14. "BRCA1 and BRCA2 Gene Mutations," KnowBRCA.org, accessed August 27, 2015, https://www.knowbrca.org/Learn/brca1-and-brca2 -gene-mutations.

15. "What are the key statistics about breast cancer?" Cancer.org, last modified June 10, 2015, accessed August 26, 2015, http://www.cancer.org/ cancer/breastcancer/detailedguide/breast-cancer-key-statistics.

16. Vincent Tuohy, "A Step Closer to Breast Cancer Vaccine," Health, Cleveland Clinic, September 17, 2013, accessed August 26, 2015, http://health. clevelandclinic.org/2013/09/a-step-closer-to-a-breast-cancer-vaccine/.

17. Lei Zehng, assistant professor of oncology and surgery at the Sidney Kimmel Comprehensive Cancer Center at Johns Hopkins University, as cited by David McNamee in "Pancreatic tumors 'reprogrammed' by new vaccine," *Medical News Today*, June 18, 2014, accessed August 26, 2015, http://www.medicalnewstoday.com/articles/278400.php.

18. Ibid.

19. "Pancreatic Cancer Vaccine," Johns Hopkins Medicine website, accessed August 26, 2015, http://www.hopkinsmedicine.org/kimmel_cancer_cen ter/centers/pancreatic_cancer/treatments/pancreatic_cancer_vaccine .html.

20. "Quick Facts," Alzheimer's Association, accessed August 26, 2015, http:// www.alz.org/facts/.

21. Doris Lambracht-Washington and Roger N. Rosenberg, "Advances in the Development of Vaccines for Alzheimer's Disease," *Discovery Medicine* 15984 (May 27, 2013): 319–326, accessed August 26, 2015, http://www .discoverymedicine.com/Doris-Lambracht-Washington/2013/05/27/ advances-in-the-development-of-vaccines-for-alzheimers-disease/.

22. Ibid.

23. David Quammen, "Stalking a Killer," *Natural Geographic*, July 2015, accessed August 26, 2015, 58.

24. Ibid., 52.

25. Ibid., 59.
26. "Safety and Biocontainment," The University of Texas Medical Branch, accessed August 26, 2015, http://www.utmb.edu/cbeid/safety.shtml.
27. "Biosafety Levels Information," Federation of American Scientists website, accessed August 26, 2015, http://fas.org/programs/bio/resource/biosafetylevels.html.
28. Alexandra Sifferlin, "Why You've Never Heard of the Vaccine for Heroin Addiction," TIME, January 9, 2015, accessed August 26, 2015, http://time.com/3654784/why-youve-never-heard-of-the-vaccine-for-heroin-addiction/.
29. George Koob, as quoted by Alexandra Sifferlin, "Why You've Never Heard of the Vaccine for Heroin Addiction," TIME, January 9, 2015, accessed August 26, 2015, http://time.com/3654784/why-youve-never-heard-of-the-vaccine-for-heroin-addiction/.
30. Kim Janda, as quoted by Alexandra Sifferlin, "Why You've Never Heard of the Vaccine for Heroin Addiction," TIME, January 9, 2015, accessed August 26, 2015, http://time.com/3654784/why-youve-never-heard-of-the-vaccine-for-heroin-addiction/.
31. Estimate based on data collected by the National Institute on Drug Abuse from the U.S. Department of Health and Human Services, Centers for Disease Control and Prevention and National Drug Intelligence Center, accessed August 26, 2015, http://www.drugabuse.gov/related-topics/trends-statistics#costs.
32. Deborah Beck, M.S.W., "Can't Get Treatment Through Your Health Insurance Plan?" HBO, accessed August 26, 2015, https://www.hbo.com/addiction/treatment/362_not_covered_by_insurance.html.
33. "Types of Vaccines," National Institute of Allergy and Infectious Diseases, accessed August 26, 2015, http://www.niaid.nih.gov/topics/vaccines/understanding/pages/typesvaccines.aspx.
34. Plotkin, "The Future of Vaccination."
35. Craig Mello during a discussion on "Re-Engineering Human Embryos," On Point, National Public Radio, April 28, 2015, accessed August 26, 2015, https://onpoint.wbur.org/2015/04/28/human-embryo-genetic-engineering-china.
36. Carl Zimmer during a discussion on "Re-Engineering Human Embryos," On Point, National Public Radio, April 28, 2015, accessed August 26, 2015, https://onpoint.wbur.org/2015/04/28/human-embryo-genetic-engineering-china.

37. Shu Ki Tsoi, Pierre R. Smeesters, Hannah R.C. Frost, Paul Licciardi and Andrew C. Steer, "Correlates of Protection for M Protein-Based Vaccines against Group A Streptococcus," *Journal of Immunology Research,* Volume 2015 (2015), Article ID 167089, accessed August 26, 2015, doi:10.1155/2015/16 7089, http://www.hindawi.com/journals/jir/2015/167089.

38. Lauran Neergaard, "Strep's evolution may provide clues for developing a vaccine," *The Associated Press,* August 10, 2015, accessed August 26, 2015, http://www.denverpost.com/nationworld/ci_28618201/nation-world -briefs-clinton-says-all-e-mails.

NOTES TO CONCLUSION

1. Gareth Williams, "From Jenner to Wakefield."

2. J. Eric Oliver and Thomas J. Wood, "Conspiracy Theories and the Paranoid Style(s) of Mass Opinion," *American Journal of Political Science*, first published online March 5, 2014, DOI: 10.1111/ajps.12084.

3. David Major, retired senior FBI supervisory special agent and first director of Counterintelligence, Intelligence and Security Programs at the National Security Council at the White House, interview with the author, June 2, 2014.

Index

Adjuvant, 107–111, 148, 171, 197
Anthrax, 6–7, 175, 197
Artificial immunity, 119–120, 197
Autism, x, 2, 5, 12, 14, 37, 56, 62,
    77–102, 107, 109, 112, 114–117,
    129, 160, 194, 197

BRCA1, 178–179, 190, 197
BRCA2, 178, 197

Carrier species, *see* Reservoir host
Case series, 79, 99–100, 198
Chickenpox (varicella), 38–39, 49,
    54, 67, 70, 89, 120, 123, 124,
    132, 146–147, 170, 198
Cohort study, 99–100, 102, 127,
    198
Conjugate vaccine, 76, 172–173,
    198

Diphtheria, 9–10, 13–14, 23,
    25–26, 48, 52, 64, 70, 89, 96,
    104, 106, 113, 128, 172, 198
DNA vaccine, 127, 173–175, 188,
    198
Double-blind study, 15, 198

DTaP, 23, 25, 27–28, 37, 39, 48, 51,
    52, 54–55, 89, 104, 113–114,
    128, 198

Edwardsiella tarda, 198
Epidemic, 71, 147, 152, 156, 167,
    181–182, 198

Formaldehyde, 104–106, 171–172,
    198

German measles (rubella), 13, 146,
    199
Guillain-Barré Syndrome, 17–18,
    199

H1N1, 73–74, 199
Hepatitis A, 8, 38, 49, 70, 89, 199
Hepatitis B, 8, 21–25, 38, 42, 52,
    64, 93, 104, 110, 172, 177, 199
Herd immunity, 13, 29, 70,
    127–128, 153, 199
Homeopathy, xi, 135–139, 141–
    144, 147, 199
Homeoprophylaxis, 135, 136, 143,
    145, 148, 199

Human papillomavirus (HPV), 47, 50, 52, 56–57, 155, 199
Humoral response, 199

Immunogenicity, 174, 199
Immunoglobulin A (IgA), 122, 199
Immunoglobulin G (IgG), 121, 200
Inactivated vaccine, 171, 200
Influenza (flu), 7, 8, 23, 25, 29, 35, 48–54, 64, 68, 70–72, 74, 89, 114, 123, 126, 128, 173, 175, 199, 200
Intussusception, 35, 40, 44–45, 200

Law of Similars, 137, 141, 143, 200
Live, attenuated vaccine, 170, 200

Measles (rubeola), ix, 4–6, 9–11, 13, 37, 48, 62, 64, 67, 70, 86, 92, 96, 99, 120, 128, 131–132, 134, 146–147, 152–153, 161, 170, 176–177, 182, 199, 200
Meningococcal disease, 11, 36–37, 128, 167, 200
MMR, ix, 6, 9, 11, 14, 23, 37–39, 48, 52, 54, 56, 61, 87, 89, 92, 94–95, 98–100, 132, 156, 194, 200
Mumps, ix, 6, 8, 9, 13, 23, 37, 48, 52, 64, 67, 70, 86, 96, 99, 120, 132, 146, 153, 170, 200

Natural immunity, 119–121, 123–126, 127, 131, 133–134, 200
Naturally acquired immunity, 119–120, 201
Nosode, 145, 148, 201
Notifiable diseases, 8, 9, 201

Oncogenic, 57, 201

Pandemic, 71, 73, 126, 201

Pertussis (whooping cough), 8, 9–10, 25, 27, 48, 55, 63-64, 75, 96, 104, 107, 113, 128, 171, 201
Phase I clinical trial, 168, 178, 183–184, 201
Phase II clinical trial, 168, 178, 201
Phase III clinical trial, 168, 178, 183–184, 201
Plasmids, 174, 201
Pneumococcal disease, 23, 25, 30–31, 36, 39, 49, 76, 174, 201
Poliovirus (polio), ix, 3–4, 10, 13–14, 17, 23, 25, 31–33, 37, 48, 50–51 52, 54, 64, 70, 73, 96, 104, 128, 134, 136, 161, 171, 201

Recombinant vector vaccine, 175–176, 202
Reservoir host, 182–183, 197, 202
Rotavirus, 23, 25, 34–35, 39–40, 45, 49, 120, 170, 188, 202

Smallpox, ix, 5–7, 11–14, 48, 63, 70, 73, 128, 169, 193, 202
Subacute Sclerosing Panencephalitis (SSPE), 5, 202
Subunit vaccine, 171–172, 202

Tetanus, 23, 25–27, 47–48, 52, 64, 70, 75, 89, 96, 104, 113, 172, 198, 202
Thimerosal, 75, 86, 89, 94, 98, 100, 101, 103, 106, 107, 111–117, 202
Toxoid, 172, 202

Vaccination, x, xi, 202
Variolation, ix, 202